Table of Contents

To my wife, Silvia, for pointing me in the low-carb/high-fat direction, having faith in me, and for walking with me along my journey of understanding weight management.

—Steve, Torino, Italy, 2020

Cover art by Andrea Holden

Forward by Steve Anthony

<u>This book is not about fat-shaming</u>. Not even close. But it's also not about ignoring the fact that as a society we are getting fatter—and being fat is not healthy. Being lean does not guarantee being healthy but getting and staying fat is associated with a host of conditions that can lead to Type 2 diabetes, heart disease, stroke, high blood pressure, and, if not causing cancer, it can certainly hide cancer symptoms and symptoms of other diseases. This book is also NOT about selling you more stuff like meal plans, special food or premium website access. There is a website for the book (**beleansecrets.com**), but it is free. It contains links to resources and a running photo log of the food Evan, and I eat.

I was fat—and am still a little overweight as I write this book. By the time I started losing weight that stayed off, I had hit 365 pounds (I'm six-feet tall). For much of my life I've experienced fat shaming and just life as a fat man. Overweight people know the looks as we walk down the aisle on an airplane and the sigh of resignation of the person assigned the seat next to ours; the looks we get at restaurants when we order the same amount of food as everyone else at the table; and the hundreds of other everyday jabs we get from the lean public. There are also logistical concerns overweight people have that lean people don't. I used to only buy slip-on shoes because bending over to tie my shoes was difficult; when climbing a big set of stairs, I'd often need to stop to catch my breath so I would pretend to be looking for something in my briefcase or backpack; when entering or leaving a restaurant, I'd need to figure out the route with the widest spaces between tables. I could go on…

I heard a random conversation on TV where a doctor said that once you hit 400 pounds, odds are you will never lose weight—because exercise becomes too hard. Those words motivated me to try to lose weight, again.

Like many of you who have picked up this book, I wasn't new to dieting and exercise. My doctor prescribed "eat less/move more" at the end of every visit. And I would give it a try. Eating less and moving more would work for a while, then stop working. Then, even while eating less and moving more, I would slowly start gaining the weight back. I blamed myself. I must have been doing something wrong… I'm sure others in my life thought the same thing.

As of writing this book (November 2019), I've lost 176 pounds. It took about four years to lose the first 100 pounds—I was using a points-based system and didn't really understand what I was doing. I had stalled in terms of weight loss and had even started to gain some of the weight back. The most recent 76 pounds have come off since January 2019. It's this experience I want to tell you about.

Some of what you are about to read will sound too good to be true—but it is true. Some of what you will read will sound unbelievable, some made me angry—angry that I was given advice that almost never works; that I struggled with my weight for nearly 50 years before finding the "long-lost secrets of weight management," and seeing how easy it is to be lean once you know these secrets. Understanding and following the information in this book has changed my life. Not just because of the weight loss. The real change is that I now know what to do to stay lean the rest of my life.

I've taken the knowledge and experience from dozens of books and research studies and condensed it into a very concise and readable format that will let you make decisions about what you eat that will let you live a lean life. I hope you find it helpful!

Me (with an Intern) in 2008
at probably 340 pounds

...and with my wife, Silvia,
at 194 pounds

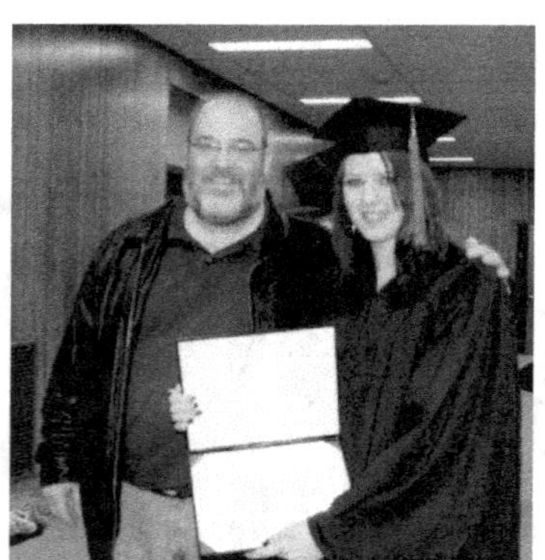

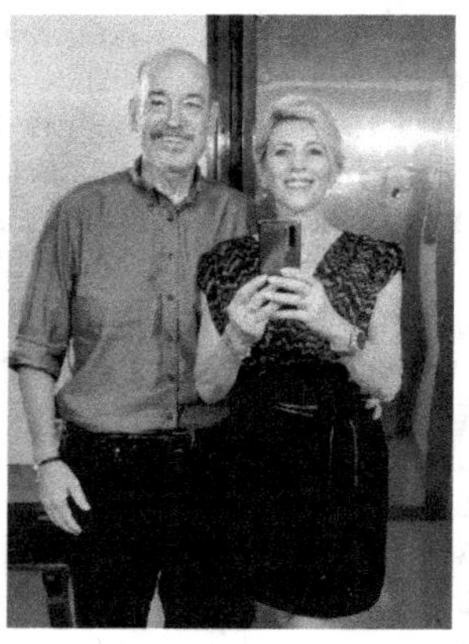

Steven Anthony, Torino, Italy

Forward by Evan Hiltunen

I was honored, and pleasantly surprised, when Steven asked me to contribute a section to this book. As a chef (ret.), and as a person that has spent almost my entire life being athletic, working out, and studying food, I have an intimate relationship with food, health, and functionality.

Many of you reading this book are doing so because you want a better understanding of why you gain weight and the best approach to losing it (in a healthy, scientifically sound manner). But, many of you with weight problems are also afflicted with other problems (like Type 2 Diabetes, cardiovascular disease, etc.). I don't have a weight problem, but I do have some special metabolic conditions that are relevant and have some of the same underlying mechanisms at play.

My own metabolic dysfunction, which I'll get into in a bit, drives my interest in this field. If I don't eat properly, I will very likely develop cardiovascular disease, fatty liver, neuropathy, very likely amputations of extremities, failing eyesight, possible blindness, certainly the kidneys will go, at some point, and I'll be on dialysis.

If I live long enough, all of those things, and more, will happen. According to my doctors.

But the fields of medicine and nutrition have been led astray from the knowledge of years past. The information contained in this book—information from as far back as 150 years ago—is somewhat shocking given how obesity and diseases like Type 2 diabetes are treated today. The good news is that many of these conditions can be reversed if they haven't progressed too far already.

As I mentioned before, I was active and athletic and measured 6' 3" and 190 lbs. Then something happened. Who knows what? But suddenly I was diagnosed with Type 2 diabetes. Now I'm listed as "surgically induced diabetes" for doctors and Type 1 for insurance; half my pancreas, all of my gallbladder, and the lower part of my stomach have been removed. I have a pancreatic duct that has scarred over (not good), IBS (alternating between diarrhea-predominant and constipation-predominant variations), and multiple bouts of pancreatitis. I need to take pills to digest my food. I inject both fast acting and long acting insulin. And even with all that, at one point, my weight plummeted to 140.

Following a diet recommended by my doctors for two years, I got my weight back up to 195 pounds, but my blood metrics were horrible! Over the summer, I switched back to a diet based on the information you will find in this book. Almost immediately my blood markers drastically improved. No one can guarantee you will get the same results, but the information revealed in this book have had a huge impact on my health and Steven's weight (I met him at his heaviest!). I hope you give it a serious try.

Evan Hiltunen, Minneapolis, Minnesota, USA

INTRODUCTION (Don't skip!)

Why is it that humans are the only self-feeding species on the planet that get overweight or obese? Sure, there are fat species like hippos, polar bears and whales. But the fat those animals have on their bodies serves a function—so while they are fat, they are not overweight. They are just as fat as they need to be to live a healthy life. The only function our *excessive* fat performs is to potentially give us Type 2 diabetes and/or a host of other ailments including heart disease.

There is an obesity epidemic in the US. Not only is the rate of being overweight or obese rising among adults (as shown here), it has also gone up among children. And obesity is on the rise world-wide.

% of US Adults 20 – 74 Classified as Obese or Extremely Obese[1]

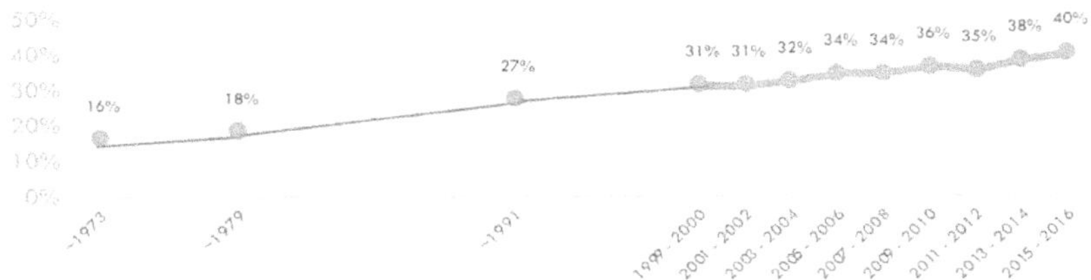

% of children 2 – 19 classified as overweight or obese [1]

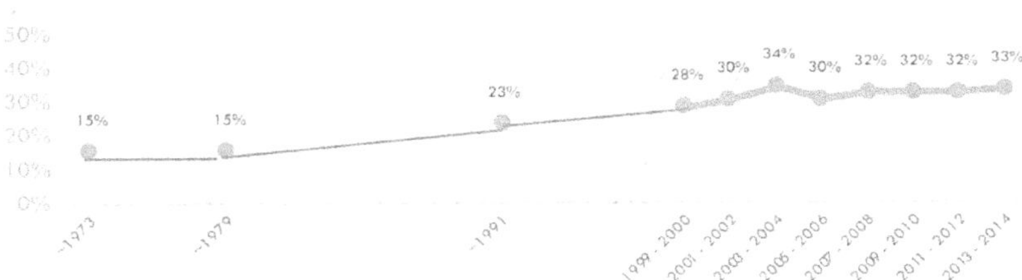

What's behind this dramatic—even alarming—increase in the excess body fat we see in modern society? It's not entirely what you think. How can you get off and/or stay off this chart and not become just another datapoint in the obesity epidemic? Again, the answer might not be what you are expecting—but **I'm confident that the information in this book will give you a better understanding of how our bodies react to the food we eat and how the types of food we eat can have a drastic impact on our weight**.

If you are overweight now, by using the information provided in this book, you will likely shed pounds like you never thought possible—I certainly did. And I did it without going hungry or joining a gym. (I'm not suggesting exercise isn't good for you—just that it has been shown not to be an effective weight-loss strategy[34].) I think you will also find it easy to keep those pounds off so you can live a healthy, lean life. If you are lean now, the information provided in this book will help you stay that way for the rest of your life.

As Americans, we have been subjects in an experiment we didn't know about. While we thought the field of nutrition and the US government were basing dietary advice and guidelines on nutritional facts, they were really telling us nutritional opinions—at best. And it turns out that many of those who told us about nutrition (our doctors, schoolteachers, parents) didn't realize that what they learned about nutrition weren't really facts. So, the good intentions of many people were misdirected by a few—who probably had our best interests in mind as well; they just failed to scientifically test their opinions to see if they were true before claiming they were true. The end result is that we've been told to follow the wrong path for a healthy diet—and the secrets of weight management became lost.

This book explains why I lost so much weight so easily—the physiology behind weight loss. But it is written for people without advanced degrees in biochemistry! Part 1 of the book covers the main things you need to know about food and how our bodies use it, so if you only read Part 1, you'll get the information you need to provide yourself (and your loved ones) a nutritious diet that will help you get and stay lean. Part 2 was written by my friend, Evan Hiltunen. In Part 2, Evan covers topics around the right attitude to have when starting a new relationship with food, food quality. At the end of the book Evan offers some simple recipes to get you going on path to being lean.

If you want to know more details about how our bodies use the food we eat or why we've been told what we've been told all these years, finish the book. I'll present a bit on these topics in Part 1 of the book, but there are more details in Part 3. In Part 4 of the book, Evan provides some tips to approaching the diet described in this book.

As you will see, this book provides you with information. Some of the information you might know already. Some will surely be new to you. Some will go against everything you have been told by your parents, your teachers and even your doctor about what goes into a healthy diet. But the information you will find here is based on scientific research and acknowledged nutritional science. That said, this is not a science text. The systems this book covers are incredibly complex and describing them in every detail is beyond the point of this book. My desire is to explain the overall way our bodies interact with the food we eat. Sometimes I oversimplify the process being described or use analogies to make it more understandable. When I do this, I give you references to resources that more fully explain the topic.

I ask that you look at the evidence—the information, the science behind what I present here. I know it is difficult to know what to believe these days: One day butter is evil, and then butter is okay to eat; cholesterol is bad, then it's just one kind of cholesterol is bad and the other is actually good. It can be confusing.

In this book, I have put an easy to understand guide on how you can judge for yourself what advice to follow and what to discard. And I've put that in an appendix so as not to get in the way of the information you need to know, or the story behind how we came to be told what we've been told.

Now that you have a copy of this book in your hands, I have no further financial interest in this topic: I don't sell meal plans or special food or t-shirts or hats. My website, **beleansecrets.com**, is free—there is no gold or platinum version to upgrade to. My goal is simply to share the information I learned that helped me lose 49% of my body weight. The only thing I have to gain now is the satisfaction that you have the information you need to make truly informed decisions about what you eat so you will live a healthy, lean life.

The website has links to resources that will help you stay on track if you are trying to lose weight. And there is a section with a bunch of photos of the things Evan and I eat—to help you get ideas of what to include in your healthy diet.

Throughout the book, there are references to specific research papers. The references are noted by little numbers in parentheses—like the "[1]" next to the title of the graphs on page 9. You can find copies of these references online and review them for yourself if you like. This is how science works: I'm providing information related to nutrition, and I'm showing you where this information comes from. You, if you are skeptical, can check the research and other sources of information I'm supplying here and check to see if my interpretation of that information is correct. The point here is that I'm not just saying "I know best, trust me!" I'm being open that the ideas I'm presenting are built on research and the expert knowledge of respected scientists in their field of science and/or medicine.

There is also a Suggested Reading List with books and links related to the topics covered here that go into much more detail and much more of the history behind the various topics. I never imagined books on nutrition could be so interesting. I strongly recommend every book on the list.

Okay—now you can get to the meat of the book!

Be prepared for some shocking news…

NOTE: The information and opinions contained in this book are not intended to represent the medical advice of physicians. The information this book presents is meant to give you information so you can make informed decisions about the food you eat. Before utilizing the dietary information presented here, you should consult your doctor. It is especially critical that you discuss this information with your doctor if you are on any medication for a chronic illness such as diabetes or epilepsy, or if you need to take insulin, other diabetes medication(s) or diuretics because changing your diet could require a change in dosage of your medication.

Be aware, however, that many doctors don't know the information presented here and have often been misled by those teaching them in med school and those in the pharmaceutical industry. See Appendix TALKING TO DOCTORS for my advice on the topic.

PART 1: OVERVIEW

Weight **gain** is a process. We don't gain 20 pounds overnight—it happens over time and can happen even if you don't overeat. In the same way, weight **loss** is a process, not an event—and simply eating less to lose weight almost never works[22].

This book will show you how the body uses the food you eat to regulate your weight. It shows how this regulation system can get knocked out of whack, and **how you can easily get it back on course, lose weight, and stay lean for life.**

Part 1 of this book covers the key information everyone needs to know to stay lean for life. When you finish Part 1, you will have a basic understanding of:

- **Nutrition**: This section reviews the nutrients found in various foods and their importance in our diet.

- **Metabolism**: This section reviews how the body reacts to and uses the nutrients we eat.

- **Why people get fat**: This section looks at the process by which many of us get fat and what likely has led to the obesity epidemic we have in the USA and around the world.

- **How to get (and stay) lean**: Combining the understanding of Nutrition, Metabolism and how we gain weight, this section describes a healthy diet and how to determine what you should and shouldn't be eating.

NUTRITION

As we look at nutrition, keep in mind that we eat for two basic reasons:
1. To get the energy we need to keep our bodies running (that is, to stay alive)
2. To get the raw materials we need to maintain our bodies (to stay healthy while alive)

It is the fact that we have these two separate, yet related, motivations behind eating that make what you eat, and when you eat it, so important.

The Basics

There are six nutrients we are likely all familiar with:
- 3 Macronutrients—things we typically eat in relatively large amounts:
  - Protein
  - Fat
  - Carbohydrates (Carbs)

- 2 micronutrient categories—things needed in relatively small amounts:
  - Vitamins (A, B-complex, C, etc.): These help the body absorb macronutrients and essential minerals as well as aiding in the creation of energy in our cells and maintaining other systems (nervous or circulatory systems, for example) in our bodies—we typically get vitamins by eating foods that contain them (we can also take supplements).
  - Minerals (Calcium, sodium, copper, etc.): Like vitamins, minerals don't provide the body with energy, but can help the body run better and keeps the various systems running well.

- Water: This is what we consume the most.

We need to eat/drink all of these things, except one, in various amounts to stay alive.

Protein

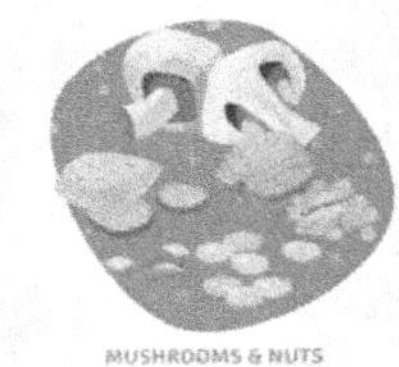

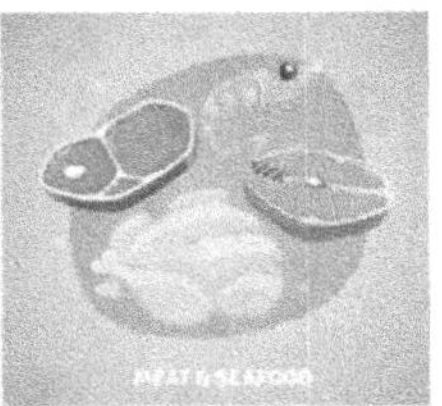

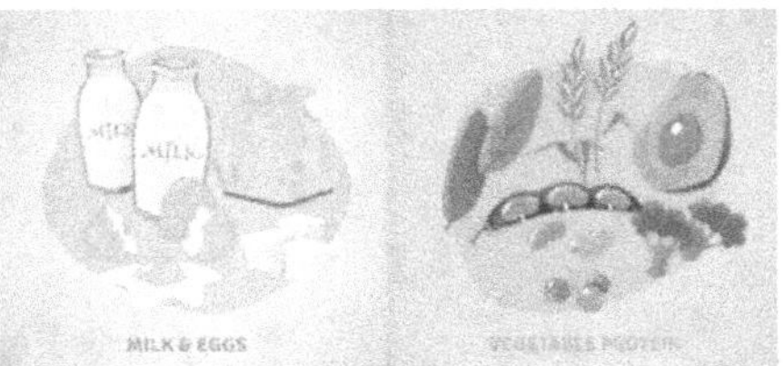

Protein is an important part of every cell in the body. Our bodies use protein to build and repair all sorts of tissue. Our bodies use protein to make enzymes, hormones, and other body chemicals as well. Protein is also used in building skin, bones, muscles, cartilage and even blood.

While our muscles are made of protein, muscle is not a form of stored protein our bodies can easily use. That is, if our bodies need protein to help mend a broken bone, it does not turn first to protein from our muscles to do it—first it looks for other protein in the body. So, to keep your body running and in good repair, you need to eat protein—and specifically 9 essential amino acids (the building blocks for proteins). We actually need 20 different amino acids, but the body will make 11 of them out of other proteins. The other 9 cannot be made by the body—that's why they are called "essential" proteins. It means it is <u>essential</u> that we <u>eat</u> them.

The good thing is you will get all 9 of your essential proteins if you eat a mix of:
- Meat: Beef, chicken, pork, fish, eggs
- Dairy: Milk, cheese
- Nuts
- Avocado

Fat

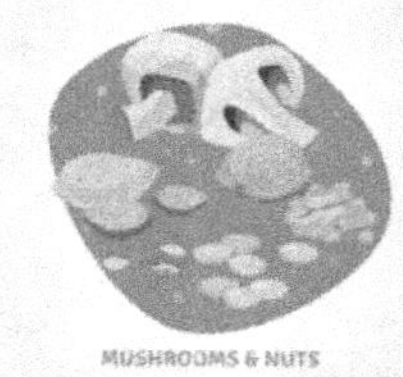
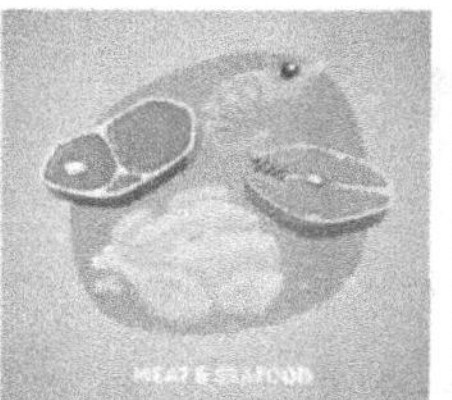
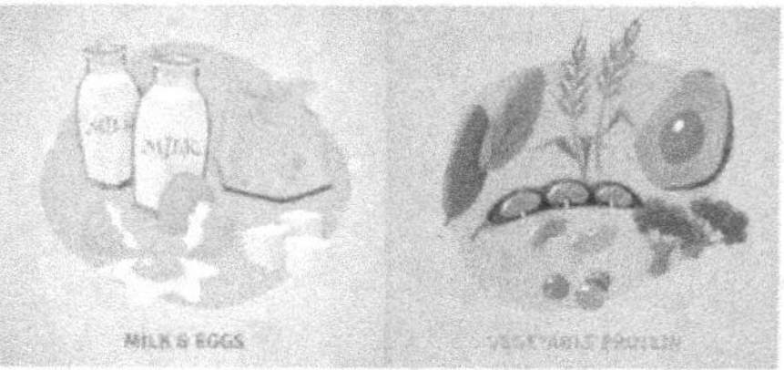

There are two types of **fat** discussed in this book: Body fat (the fat we store in our bodies) and dietary fat (the fat we eat). And no, the illustration is not a mistake—it's just that fats are often found in foods with protein.

Dietary fat comes in different types:
- Saturated fat—typically the fat found in animal products (meat, fish, full-fat dairy)
- Unsaturated fat, which comes in two types:
  - Monounsaturated—like the kind you get from extra virgin olive oil
  - Polyunsaturated—like the kind you get from corn oil and other seed oils
- Trans fats/Hydrogenated fats—often found in highly processed foods and fast food

There are 2 essential fatty acids (scientific term for fats) and you've probably heard of those recently—omega-3 and omega-6. You often see in the news that omega-6 is bad and that omega-3 is good. But in reality, we need both—both are **essential** fatty acids. The problem with omega-6 is that we tend to get too much of it in our diet and not enough omega-3. Some foods, like chicken, have both omega-3 and omega-6, so we get both from one food, and in healthy amounts (if you leave the skin on). Where our typical diets give us too much omega-6 is from the use of polyunsaturated oils, especially seed oils, we were encouraged to eat—like corn, soybean, sunflower and cottonseed oil. Cutting these oils from your diet and using cold-pressed extra virgin olive oil will go a long way lowering your levels of omega-6. A lot of processed foods also contain polyunsaturated oils. So, avoiding highly processed foods can help reduce the amount of omega-6 from the diet.

Why we were told to use seed oils is rather unbelievable and discussed in Appendix ONE MAN'S EGO. **Body fat** comes from the food we eat—but not directly.

Both dietary and body fat can play an important role in brain development, cell growth, the physical protection of organs (think airbags) and insulation for the body.

Carbohydrates

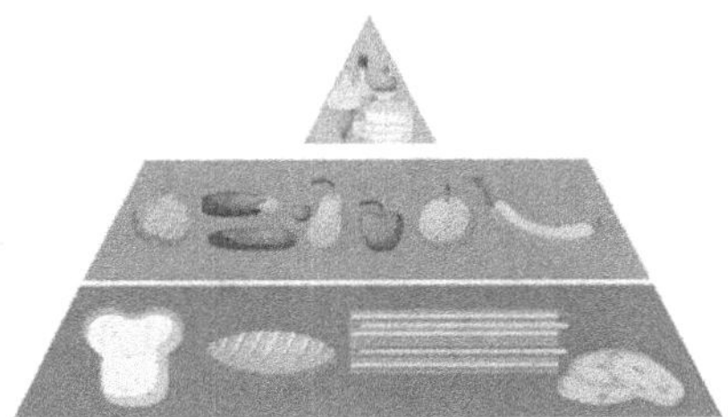

Unlike protein and fat, there are **no essential carbohydrates**. We could live our entire lives without eating a single smidgeon of carbs. Some might question the quality of such a life! But after reading this book, you will likely agree that a reduction in how many carbs we eat might be worth considering. As you might guess from the illustration, carbs are the base of our current recommended diet as depicted by the familiar food pyramid—and also at the tip of the food pyramid.

*Side Note: This is an area many doctors and nutritionists will object to. They will point to the fact that the brain needs glucose (blood sugar) to function and we get glucose from the carbohydrates we eat. Some will go on to say since the brain needs an estimated 480 calories a day, and carbohydrates provide 4 calories per gram, that we need to eat at a minimum about 120 grams of carbs a day. That's the equivalent of about half a pound of sugar (only half of table sugar gets broken down into glucose)! Granted it doesn't need to be table sugar—bread, pasta, rice, potatoes all contain carbohydrates which get converted to glucose. But it's still a lot! While the brain does use carbohydrates, **if we don't eat any food that can be converted to glucose our liver will create glucose out of our stored fat** in a process called "gluconeogenesis"— which is Greek for "newly created glucose."*

The king of carbs is sugar. The sugar you find in packets at the coffee shop or in the sugar you have at home is called sucrose and is made up of glucose and fructose. Fructose is also found in fruit and in some vegetables.

Sugar is used a lot by manufacturers in their processed foods. They use sugar for a few reasons:
- If they remove fat from a product (everyone is looking for low-fat foods), it's difficult (and expensive) to replace the fat with protein—it's easy and cheap to replace the fat with sugar
- People buy more of the product if it has a lot of sugar in it
- The products with a lot of sugar have longer shelf-lives

Food manufacturers know that our conscious minds also want foods without so much sugar (even though our pleasure centers will guide us to buy the product that tastes sweeter). Because of this, manufacturers show sugar on the ingredient labels in some not-so-familiar ways. A few examples of sugars that sound healthy are honey, maple syrup and agave nectar. Some that don't sound sweet at all include barley malt, maltodextrin, diatase and dextran. Manufacturers often use a mix of sugars in their products so "sugar" doesn't end up first (or high up) on the ingredient list!

Carbs can also be described as being unrefined (I like the term "natural") or refined (I like the term "processed"). <u>Natural carbs</u> are the ones you can eat without doing anything except washing (and maybe peeling) them—like fruits and vegetables. In moderation, fruits and vegetables have a place in most meal plans. Later in the book, how to judge what "moderation" means for you is discussed.

Some natural carbs include things like:
- Potatoes
- Nuts
- Seeds
- Vegetables
- Fruit

<u>Processed carbs</u>, like bleached (white) rice, refined flour, High Fructose Corn Syrup and many of the sugars listed above are everywhere in processed foods.

Some foods containing processed carbs include things like:
- Bread
- Cereal
- Pasta
- Salad dressing
- Candy

Most carbs get broken down into glucose (a form of sugar) in your digestive tract. Even though the body keeps just over 1 teaspoon of glucose in the blood, you don't need to eat any carbs to get that glucose. Why? Because if there isn't enough glucose coming into our bodies from the food we eat, our liver will make it out of fat in our body. That's right! Our bodies will take body fat and convert it to glucose if we don't eat enough carbs to supply the body what it needs. That's why there are no "essential dietary carbohydrates."

The big problem with processed carbs is that they get digested early in the digestive system, before they can trigger signals to the brain that you are full. At mealtime, my mother always used to tell me not to fill up on bread—apparently when she was young, she would get full by eating too much bread. But I always thought "I don't get full from eating bread!" This speaks to how even refined carbohydrates have changed over time—becoming even more processed/refined. This change has also likely contributed to the obesity epidemic (see Appendix THE CASE AGAINST PROCESSED CARBS).

Natural carbs stay in your digestive system longer and can trigger signals of being full.

The biggest problem with carbohydrates is that they trigger our pancreas to put insulin in our blood—which brings us to the topic of Metabolism.

Side Note: Some fruits and vegetables have been bred to contain more sugar— just look at the different types of apples there are and how sweet some of them are. The University of Minnesota has developed many of the apples you find in the supermarket today. On their apple website, they describe developing sweeter apples. Sweeter apples have a longer freshness window and people like them more. So sweeter apples are good for business—but not necessarily your health.

In the late 1950s, two biochemists (Richard O. Marshall and Earl R. Kooi) discovered a way to convert the sucrose in corn syrup into a very dense form of fructose that was later called High Fructose Corn Syrup. In the 1970s, HFCS was introduced in the food industry as a much cheaper form of sweetener. Today you can see High Fructose Corn Syrup (often just listed as HFCS) in many of the processed foods available in the US and around the world. You can even find High Fructose Corn Syrup in foods you wouldn't think would have sugar (which is what HFCS is) in them like: Frozen pizza, many yogurts, salad dressings, bread, boxed dinners like macaroni and cheese, nutrition bars, sports drinks and even coffee creamer.

🔎 Key Points to Remember:

- There are three macronutrients
  - Protein
  - Fat
  - Carbohydrates
- There are essential proteins and essential fats, but there are NO essential carbohydrates
- If we don't take in enough carbohydrates to supply the brain with the glucose it needs, the liver will create glucose from our stored fat by a process called gluconeogenesis.
- Processed food can contain much more sugar that we realize
- Some manufacturers try to mislead you about how much sugar is in their products by using small amounts of many different sugars—some of which don't sound sweet at all.

METABOLISM

The dictionary defines metabolism as the chemical processes that occur in the body in order to keep it alive. It's what our bodies do to convert the food we eat to the energy we need to live and to maintain our bodies. It's something our bodies do without our conscious direction—we don't tell our bodies to digest food and to convert it to energy; the body just does it. This definition links back to the two reasons we eat listed at the beginning of the Nutrition section of the book.

When it comes to the primary sources of energy to live on, the body can use either glucose or fat. It's as if our life engine can use either gasoline or diesel—whichever is available. Our metabolic processes make and store both fuels in our body, and it has a strict set of rules of when it uses each—and it can only use one primary fuel at a time.

As you can probably tell already, metabolism in the human body is incredibly complex—and describing it fully is beyond the scope of this book. What is provided here is a basic explanation of what happens to the food we eat after we eat it, focusing on the main process of generating energy from that food and using the energy produced to live our lives. (A good source for details on metabolism is: Human Metabolism: A Regulatory Perspective by Keith N. Frayn and Rhys Evans.)

Before we get into how we metabolize food, however, it will help to look at how our ancient ancestors lived and ate, as this will give us clues as to how our metabolic systems came to be the way they are today.

An important thing to keep in mind here is that we evolved from our ancient ancestors over millions of years. The food available back then, and over time, was much different than it is today. For example, it was only just over 12,000 years ago that people started cultivating grains and other foods to eat. Prior to that, we were mostly "hunter-gatherers."

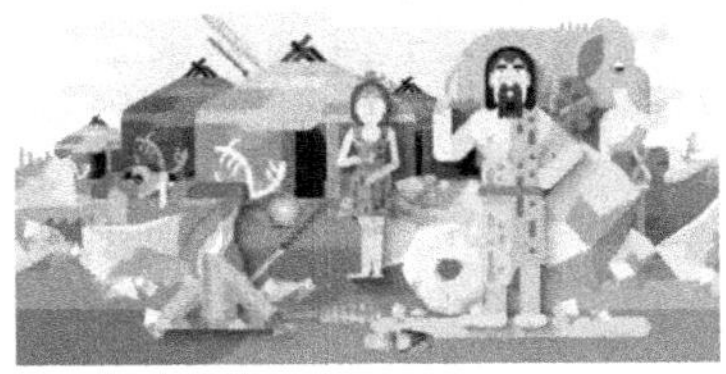

As the name suggests, hunter-gatherers got food from either hunting it (deer, buffalo, etc.) or gathering it (fruit, nuts, seeds, vegetables) when they came across it. Hunting resulted in protein and fat. Gathering resulted in carbohydrates (there is also some proteins and fats in those gathered foods, but they're largely carbs). The fruits and vegetables gathered were typically what could be found above ground—fruits and leafy plants that have relatively few carbs. We, and our way of metabolizing food, evolved based on eating a lot of protein and fat, with some carbohydrates.

Storing fat is thought to have given us a couple of advantages over animals that don't store much fat[20]. An average lean, healthy, human male is between 12% and 20% body fat. At 150 pounds, that man would have enough fat to last a month or more without eating any food. This allowed us to roam farther from a food source to find other sources of food. By contrast, male Chimps, for example, are only about 0.005% body fat; they can't stray very far for risk of not finding enough food. Storing fat over building muscle also allowed our brains to get bigger—both muscle and brain tissue use a lot of energy, so you can't have a lot of both.

Evolutionary changes can take tens of thousands of generations to occur—with genetic changes getting passed down from parents to children. Anthropologists consider a new generation every 20 years. So, even though 12,000 years of cultivating crops seems like a long time, it has only been about 600 generations. Our ancestors were evolving as hunter-gatherers for 2,300,000 years—115,000 generations. In generational terms, cultivated grains (and more recently, processed foods) have NOT been part of our diet for 99.995% of human history.

🔎 Key Points to Remember:
- Metabolism is the process that converts the food we eat into nutrients our bodies can use for energy and maintenance.
- We can use glucose or fat for fuel—but there are strict rules over which one we use at a given time.
- Our metabolism evolved over a long period of time. During this evolution, our ancient ancestors had a lot of access to protein and fat—but not so much access to carbohydrates.
- We humans, and our metabolic process, have spent 99.995% of our time on earth without access to cultivated crops that are high in carbohydrates.

Building Blocks

As we delve further into metabolism, it might help to think of our metabolism like someone building a house. The builder needs certain materials like bricks, wooden beams, plastic pipes, metal nails and glass windows to build the house. Like the builder, we need certain materials to build and maintain our bodies. But there is a difference between our metabolism and the builder. The builder can <u>buy</u> bricks, wooden beams, plastic pipes, metal nails and glass windows to build the house from a store; we have to make all our building materials ourselves—from the food we <u>eat</u>.

As you will see, metabolism is a process that <u>breaks down</u> the food we eat into the most basic raw materials, <u>makes</u> things we need from those raw materials, and then <u>breaks down</u> those things we made to give us energy (now or later) or maintain our bodies. Our bodies need energy to survive—and we can't convert a cheeseburger directly into energy. The body needs to break down the food we eat and build the basic raw materials of glucose (from carbs), amino acids (from protein) and fatty acids (from fat). The body can then use these basic raw materials to produce energy.

Before we go on to what happens when we eat, consider this: Aside from the role your parents played in creating you, you exist because of the food you eat. Everything that is you right now, started as food: You ate food, your metabolic system took that food and broke it down to molecules of glucose (from carbs), amino acids (from proteins) and fatty acids (from fats), and then your body fueled itself with glucose (and something else that will be discussed later) and kept it running with the amino and fatty acids. It really is true that we are what we eat.

With that in mind, we will move on to how the food we eat becomes part of us.

What Happens When We Eat

The purpose of our metabolic process is to provide us with energy to live and the "building" materials to keep our bodies healthy while we are alive.

Our metabolic process perks up even before we eat—it starts up when we see, smell or even think of food. We can start to get hungry (or hungrier) when any of those things happen. That's why grocery stores often make you walk through the baked-goods section (wonderful smells) or the produce section (beautiful

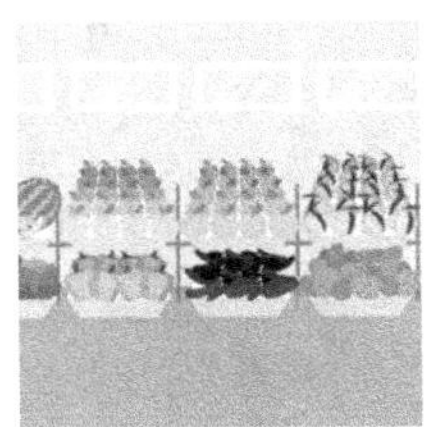

displays of colorful fruits and vegetables) when you first enter the store. These sections get you hungry and likely to buy more. You might have gotten a little hungry just reading this paragraph!

Digestion: But the real meat (pun intended) of the process of metabolism starts when we put food into our **digestive system**—that is, when we eat.

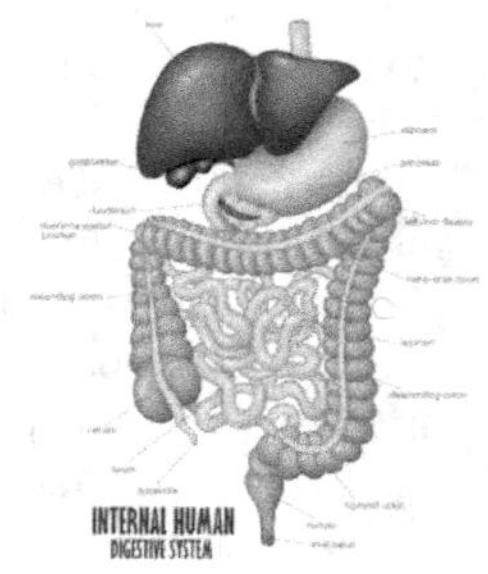

The food we put in our mouths interacts with our saliva and along with the act of chewing, starts to break down the food into raw materials our bodies can use to build the materials it needs for energy and maintenance. The stomach and small intestine continue this process of breaking down food. They break the food down into its basic building blocks, which depend on the type of nutrient it is. This was an incredibly simplistic description of the digestive system, but complete enough for the purposes of this book—the food we eat gets broken down into its basic component nutrients, that then get absorbed and used by our bodies.

Proteins get broken down into amino acids—remember, we have 9 essential amino acids. There are 11 other amino acids our bodies need, but our bodies can make those out of other nutrients if need be. The 9 essential ones can't be made by the body, which is why it's **essential** that we eat them.

Fats get broken down into fatty acids—they can also be called lipids. These fatty acids take the form of glycerides, triglycerides and cholesterol. You've probably heard of triglycerides in ads for certain drugs on TV or your doctor might have discussed them with you when reviewing a blood test. There are only 2 essential fatty acids— omega-3 and omega-6.

Carbohydrates get broken down mainly into glucose. Carbohydrates in the form of fiber don't get broken down into anything and aren't used directly by the body. Fiber is thought, however, to help feed the bacteria in our gut that helps us digest food, among other things. If you eat sucrose (table sugar), that is broken down into glucose and fructose.

Fructose bypasses the path glucose takes (described a bit later) and will be stored as fat in the liver; if the liver is full, it will be stored as fat elsewhere in the body.

After being broken down to basic components, these components are absorbed into the body in the stomach, small intestine or large intestine.

<u>Amino acids</u>:   Once in the bloodstream, amino acids are used for building/maintaining cells, making hormones, and a host of other things. Amino acids are not typically used for fuel unless all other sources of energy in the body are gone.

<u>Blood-lipids</u> (fat in the blood): When we eat fat, the fatty acids (lipids) get stored as body fat or used as fuel for cells, depending on the set of strict rules mentioned earlier (the specific rules will be discussed shortly).

<u>Blood sugar</u>: When glucose enters the blood stream, we refer to it as blood glucose, or, blood sugar. You often hear diabetics talk about what their blood sugar or blood glucose levels are. Normal blood glucose levels are between 70 and 100 mg/dL (milligrams per deciliter) when fasted (not eaten overnight)—it can get up to 180 mg/dL after eating, especially if you've just eaten a lot of carbs. People sometimes get cranky ("hangry") when they haven't eaten, and their blood sugar gets low (maybe down to 60 mg/dL). If your blood sugar gets extremely low, you can faint, have a seizure (around 20 mg/dL) or go into a coma (under 20 mg/dL). There is danger if your blood glucose levels get too high as well.

As you can probably tell, while we typically love the taste of sugar, our bodies have a love/hate relationship with it. Glucose (the words glucose and sugar will be used interchangeably here) provides cells with a quick form of energy. But too much glucose can lead to death—but it doesn't typically kill you quickly. If you consistently have high levels of blood sugar, like Type 2 diabetics do, the excess glucose can cause nerve damage and blood circulation damage. The circulation system damage can lead to blindness, kidney failure and limb amputation. High blood glucose levels have also been linked to heart disease. But this happens over decades.

Our Metabolic OS

Like most of our operating systems (body temperature, for example), our bodies like to keep just the right amount of glucose in the blood—not too little and not too much. In our 5 liters of blood (in an adult body) that equates to about 5 grams of glucose (just over a teaspoon); for an 80-pound child, it's about half that amount—2.6 grams (about half a teaspoon), because they have less blood. As mentioned above, the body does allow for a "plus or minus" range around that target. Damage, however, can be done if the blood sugar level gets over that upper range so our bodies try to keep that amount of glucose relatively constant. It has a few ways to store that glucose which will be discussed a bit later.

One of the problems with high blood sugar is that there are really no easily seen symptoms of it. Gaining weight is one sign, but in children, it's difficult to know if it's just part of a growth spurt or real weight gain. And the weight gain for an adult can be ounces per year—but over 20 or 30 years, it adds up to obesity and, potentially, Type 2 diabetes.

While proteins and fats do play a role in blood sugar levels, their role is much, much smaller than the role of carbohydrates—and especially sugar.

Key Points to Remember:
- Our metabolic process breaks down the food we eat into the basic stuff our bodies can use to power (glucose and fatty acids) and maintain itself (protein).
- Proteins and fats are broken down into essential amino and fatty acids.
- Carbohydrates get broken down mainly into glucose.
- Glucose levels in the blood need to stay within a safe range or it can damage the body.
- Type 2 diabetes is a condition where the body has trouble using glucose.

How the Body Deals with Carbohydrates

<u>Insulin</u>: There are many hormones (chemical signals in the body) that deal with metabolism, but the one that probably plays the biggest role when it comes to managing blood glucose is insulin. You've likely heard of insulin before—it's what many Type 2 diabetics need to inject themselves with to control their blood sugar levels because the insulin they produce doesn't do the job. Type 1 diabetics need to inject insulin because their body doesn't produce ANY insulin. Insulin has many jobs within the body and managing blood sugar levels is a big one.

When we eat and start to digest carbohydrates, signals are sent from the mouth and stomach to the pancreas to start pumping insulin into the blood stream. When the carbs are broken down and glucose is absorbed into the blood, it is the insulin that takes it through our bodies.

The first thing insulin will do is offer the glucose to our cells for energy. Each of our cells can store a bit of glucose for use. And each cell has a door of sorts, with a bouncer in front, that recognizes insulin and lets the insulin know if the cell can use some glucose or if it is full for the time being. If the cell has room for some glucose, the bouncer opens the door and lets some glucose in; if the cell is full, the bouncer tells insulin to move on. 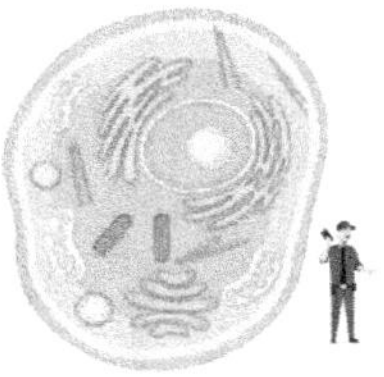

If all our cells have their fill, insulin transports the glucose to the liver. The liver converts the glucose into a denser form of sugar called glycogen. Glycogen is easily converted back into glucose. After the liver makes glycogen out of the glucose, insulin takes it to the muscles and offers it to muscle cells for storage. A similar door and bouncer system applies to glycogen and the muscle cells. If the muscle cells 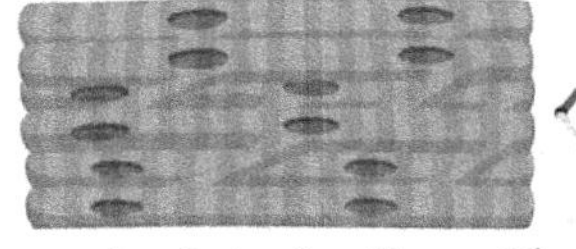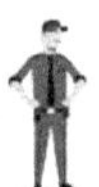 have all the glycogen they can store, the glycogen goes back to the liver. The liver itself can store some glycogen and will convert it quickly into glucose if the body needs a quick burst of energy.

If all the working cells in our bodies have enough glucose and glycogen, the extra glycogen gets converted to fat and stored in the fat cells in our body. Fat cells have doors like the other cells, but no bouncer to say, "we're full." Fat cells do have a bouncer, but their bouncer guards the <u>exit</u> of the fat cell and controls what leaves.

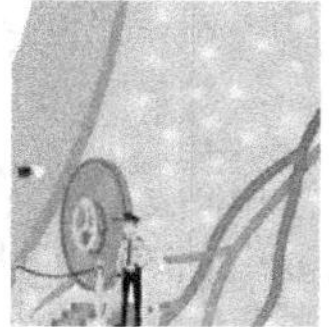

All this carting of glucose and glycogen back and forth takes time. And all that time, the extra sugar in the blood—or possibly the extra insulin itself—is damaging tissue in the body. It's a slow, but steady, process.

Insulin, then, plays a role in why we get fat—an overflow of sugar in the blood will get put into fat cells by insulin. But it gets worse: When insulin levels are high (we'll discuss how this happens next) insulin shuts down the ability of the body to take fat out of fat cells and use it for fuel. In a sense, when insulin is carting glucose around, it tells the bouncers of the fat cells to "lock it down—don't let anything out!" Thanks a lot, insulin!

But it's not that insulin hates us or wants to make us obese. The role of insulin is to reduce the amount of sugar in our blood because, as we saw, too much sugar in our blood causes damage to the body. Insulin just responds to the food we eat and does its job in the only way it can. If we eat and our blood sugar gets too high, we are going to start storing fat rather than continue to damage other tissue in our bodies because of a high level of blood sugar. It's a built-in safety system to keep the right balance of glucose in our blood—and it works just fine if we don't overdo it on the carbs.

<u>Glucagon</u>: Glucagon is a hormone related to metabolism that you probably haven't heard of before. Like insulin, glucagon is made in the pancreas. Glucagon's job is to help convert fat (both dietary and body fat) into energy for the body to use. But insulin and glucagon have a sort of chain of command they follow. This chain of command deals with which fuel we use (glucose or fat). In this chain of command insulin calls the shots—I think because it needs to be able to freely respond to an "overdose" of glucose and get it out of the blood. So, this is the strict rule: Glucagon can only do its job of getting the body to burn fat as fuel when insulin levels in the blood are relatively low. The exact relationship between insulin and glucagon is still in its early stages of research and understanding—but this seems to be how it works.

- Insulin is the hormone (most) responsible to transporting glucose around the body.
- Insulin does a lot of work to keep blood sugar at a level that is safe for the body.
- When there is a lot of insulin in the body, the body will only store fat—it will not use fat for fuel when insulin levels are high.
- Glucagon is the hormone (most) responsible for using fat for fuel.
- The ability of glucagon to burn fat for fuel depends on the level of insulin in our blood: If insulin is high, glucagon will not be allowed to burn fat.

Does the Body Prefer to Burn Glucose or Fat?

Some people in the field of nutrition see this dominance of insulin as evidence that the body prefers to burn glucose over fat. I see this a bit differently. Consider you have a fireplace. You have a big supply of firewood next to the garage (body fat) and a small supply in the den, near the fireplace (fat stored in the liver). Now, someone brings a bunch of oil-soaked rags and plops them in the middle of the den (a bunch of sugar you just ate). Personally, I'd prefer to burn the firewood—but I would burn up the oily rags first because they are dangerous.

I think the body takes this same approach with its fuel options. I think the body prefers to burn fat, but when a dangerous level of glucose enters the bloodstream, it tries to burn it up before it does too much damage.

Consider fuel preference in the context of our evolution:
1. Our ancient ancestors didn't have a lot of access to carbohydrates. Why would our bodies have evolved to prefer a fuel source that was not very plentiful?
2. Our ancient ancestors did have a lot of access to fat. Why would we have evolved in a way that didn't take advantage of this fuel source which our bodies are good at storing?
3. Anthropologists tell us that long ago, people didn't eat three meals a day—or even every day, or even every week. There was generally enough food to be found but eating just wasn't an everyday thing. Our body can store vast supplies of potential fuel as fat—enough for even a lean person to live comfortably for a few weeks without eating anything (It's estimated that body fat has about 3,500 calories per pound. Even a lean 150-pound adult

with 10% body fat has 15 pounds of fat in and around his/her body. At a daily calorie intake of 2000/day, 15 pounds of fat would provide him/her with fuel for 26 days without eating anything else.)

4. Our body can store a relatively small amount of potential energy as glucose or glycogen (the dense form of glucose)—only between 8 - 24 hours' worth.
5. While our bodies maintain a level of glucose in the blood, it can do so without the use of dietary (eaten) carbohydrates.

Back, say, 500,000 years ago, when our ancient ancestors found and gathered carbohydrates (fruits and vegetables), they ate them up and got a little fatter in the process. But this happened seasonally—they didn't have apples or oranges or tomatoes all year round. They would eat fruits and vegetables when they were available and ripe. They'd gain some fat, but they would soon use that fat for fuel.

Fasting has recently become popular. But it really just mimics the way life was for our ancient ancestors who didn't eat every day. Fasting is discussed in the Adults Only section of the book but a couple of things of note are:

- For our ancient ancestors, a life of fasting (that is, not eating every day) was not likely a life of constant fear of starvation. It was likely just how they lived based on the availability of the types of food they ate. When I started fasting as part of my approach to nutrition, I stopped what had been a constant focus on food: I no longer thought about what to eat for dinner while eating lunch, and sometimes "mealtime" would pass unnoticed because I just wasn't hungry.

- Once you've gotten out of the habit of eating three times a day (or more) or even every day, you'll find you stop getting regular hunger pangs and a growling stomach. Those signals to eat are based on your body's dependence (not necessarily preference) for glucose. These "I need more glucose" signals stop when your body switches to burning fat—because even lean people have plenty of fat to use as fuel. As mentioned earlier, carrying fat on our bodies gives us protection from a shortage of food. It's like carrying an extra battery for your phone in case it runs low on power and you can't get to an outlet.

🔑 Key Points to Remember:

- It is unclear which type of fuel our body prefers: glucose or fat
- An argument can be made that from the context of natural selection, our bodies evolved with a preference to burn fat.
- When you burn fat for fuel, you don't get the frequent signals that you are hungry.

WHY DO PEOPLE GET FAT?

Side Note: Our weight is influenced by many factors—a major one of which is the food we eat. In addition to what we eat, other important factors include: the amount of stress in our lives (less is better), the amount of sleep we get (more is better), how much alcohol we drink (less is better), family history/genetic factors and certain medical conditions.

Why Do We Gain Weight?

By understanding how our bodies **gain** weight, we can begin to look at effective ways to **lose** weight.

The amount of carbohydrates we eat, and when we eat them, has a huge impact on our weight—or at least the weight of many people. The type of carbohydrates also plays an important role in weight control.

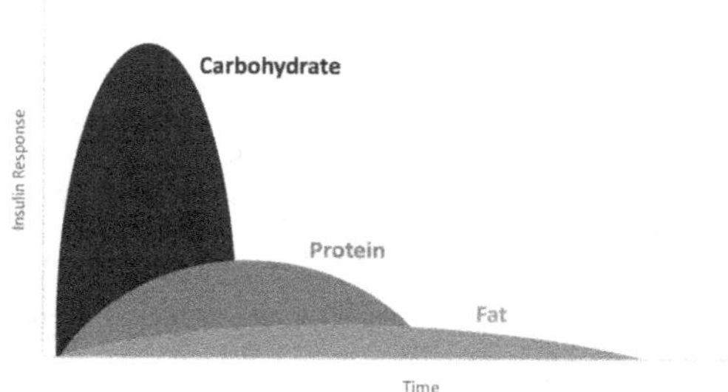

Society tells us that people get fat because they eat too much and/or don't get enough exercise. I'm sure some people get fat for those reasons. But many fat people just ate the recommended number of calories and followed the recommended (USDA) dietary guidelines in terms of what to eat.

We have seen how our bodies react to glucose in the blood. Now we'll look at how nutrition and metabolism work in a little more detail.

Insulin: The amount of insulin our pancreas puts into the blood differs depending on the macronutrient we eat (see Appendix INSULIN for more details). As you can see above, carbohydrates add the greatest amount of insulin into the bloodstream—and even different types of carbohydrates add more or less insulin to the blood. Protein

32

can add some insulin and fat, almost none. In fact, pure fat won't cause the pancreas to secrete any insulin into the blood—but it's hard to find a fat that doesn't have a little protein stuck to it.

Both the height of the insulin spike and how long it lasts are important in terms of what, and when, we eat. Of course, when we eat a mixture of macronutrients, insulin will be raised to meet the highest need. So, if we eat a lot of carbs with our meal, the pancreas will pump out enough insulin for the body to manage all the glucose contained in the meal.

Here's how a typical day might look to your pancreas if you eat a typical American diet (what is often referred to as "The Standard American Diet"):

Morning

If you eat a lot of carbs at breakfast (like a bowl of cereal with a banana on top) you will add a heavy dose of glucose to your blood (both the cereal and the banana are high in carbs). So, you will have insulin being pumped out of your pancreas from say 7:45 AM to 10:15 AM to deal with the glucose you've added to your blood. After your carby breakfast, you get a little sugar crash mid-morning and have a snack to tide you over until lunch. Let's say you are trying to be healthy, so you eat a piece of fruit—so just as your pancreas is slowing insulin production down, it gets kicked into high gear to handle the big spike in blood sugar from the carbs in your snack. The fruit holds you (but not really…) until maybe 11:30 AM, but even though your appetite is building, you hold on until lunch.

Lunch

Even if you don't eat a bit extra because you are so hungry, after an hour of rest, your pancreas is pumping out insulin again. If breakfast and snack are a daily morning routine, your pancreas has been working the whole time—which I'll explain in a bit. But lunch means more carbs at noon. More pumping insulin for the pancreas.

Afternoon Snack

Now it's sleepy-time—2:30 PM. Let's say you are trying to keep it low-fat, so you opt for pretzels instead of chips, and a diet soda instead of a regular—might as well have a zero-calorie drink. More carbs via the pretzels so more insulin. And while the zero-calorie drink has, as it says, zero calories, some artificial sweeteners causes an insulin spike as severe as, if not more so, than would the plain, regular sugared version of the drink[11]—even if having no effect on levels of blood sugar!

Dinner

You've had some time since your afternoon snack, but you wait until dinner to eat again. So maybe your pancreas has had a little break. But it's back to pumping insulin at just after 6:00 PM.

Bedtime

Even if you don't end up having an evening snack, your pancreas has had a workout dealing with all the glucose you ingested. It still might be working on the last of the excess glucose in your blood as you drift off to sleep.

Now, remember, all the while your pancreas was pumping out insulin to deal with what you ate, your body was not able to use any (or at least not very much) of its stored fat for fuel. And in addition, insulin was driving even more fat into your fat cells while you were eating and even after you ate. This fat came from any glucose that was converted to fat and from any dietary fat you ate. Your body was storing fat until your insulin level fell low enough for glucagon to start the fat-burning process—but your insulin level never dropped low enough, because of all the glucose in your blood and the insulin needed to manage it. And, again, it's not that insulin is being mean—it's trying to save your life from too much glucose in the only way it can.

If you are eating high carb meals and snacks every day (and in this context, sodas and fruit-juice count as carbohydrates!) it can cause you to become what's called "insulin resistant." Using the door and bouncer analogy, being insulin resistant is like needing more and more insulin before the bouncer recognizes it's even there. When this happens, your pancreas needs to produce even more insulin to get your cells to accept the glucose it needs. With more insulin in the blood, it takes longer for insulin levels to go down enough to allow your body to release and burn some of the fat it has been storing. It can get to the point where even during the night, insulin levels are at a high-enough level to prevent the hormone glucagon from promoting the use stored fat to fuel us while we sleep. When this happens, we might overeat in the morning because we are so hungry. Or worse, we wake up in the middle of the night for a snack.

- Our insulin response to food depends on the macronutrient content of the food.
- Carbohydrates create the biggest insulin response.
- Eating lots of carbs and snacks between meals keeps insulin levels high—possibly too high for glucagon to start the fat-burning process.
- If glucagon can't do its job, we will only store fat (not burn it).

If you've ever been overweight, your doctor will surely have told you to cut back on your food intake and get more exercise. And that seems reasonable, unless you know a lot about how the body responds to various macronutrients (which many doctors don't) or how our body responds to caloric restriction (which many doctors don't). In fact, one of the top medical school texts[3] teaches soon-to-be doctors that people get fat because they eat too much and move too little. So, doctors are just giving advice based on what they've learned.

But what about the sudden rise in obesity rates seen in the late 70s and that continue today? If we are to believe what's taught in medical schools, the implication is that starting in the late 1970s, people in the US suddenly decided to not care if they became obese. That implication needs, then, to be assumed about people around the globe as they start to follow the standard diet recommended by the US government.

There is evidence[28][29], however, that the relationship between how much we eat/move and how much we weigh goes the other way around—that overweight people *seem* to overeat and/or lead a sedentary lifestyle because they've gotten fat. So, let's look at how many people get fat.

As we saw:
- Eating a lot of carbohydrates leads to increased insulin levels—and, as we'll see later, this can easily happen if you stick to the USDA recommended amount of carbs, even on a diet based on a healthy number of calories per day
- Increased insulin levels lead to the storage of some of the food we eat (after being converted to fat by the liver) in our fat deposits
- High levels of insulin prevent the use of dietary and body fat as fuel

Eating a lot of carbohydrates each day (like the USDA guidelines suggest) can lead the body to get resistant (desensitized) to insulin, causing the body to raise levels of the hormone even higher. When this happens, the level of insulin in the blood can remain high enough all day and prevent the use of body fat for fuel during the day. This means the individual just continues to get fatter and fatter—even if they cut back on how much they eat.

Above, I said overweight people "seem to overeat." The reason "seem" is appropriate is because from the perspective of the overweight person's automatic weight control system, they are not overeating. Think about it. Let's use an example of an overweight man, who, to maintain weight (neither lose nor gain) should eat 2000 calories a day. The overweight person, with high levels of insulin, stores a percentage of everything they eat as body fat—because when following the USDA recommended diet there just isn't a way to use or store all the glucose. And, because their insulin levels are so high, glucagon can't do its job and therefore, they can never use this body fat. Let's say, for the sake of this example, that 20% of all the calories this person eats goes into fat storage.

If they stick to their 2,000 calorie/day diet, 400 calories (20% of 2000 = 400) will be sent to fat storage. That means their body can only use 1,600 calories of the 2,000 they eat for energy. This leaves the person hungry—so they eat a bit more. To us, it seems like they are overeating. But to their body, what we see as "extra food" is just what is needed to reach the 2000 calories their body needs. To get those "lost" 400 calories, they would have to eat an additional 500 calories—because 20% of the additional calories they ate would be stored as fat. The body might also try to "make up" those missing calories by getting the person to only use up 1,600 calories a day— so they look lazy. Either way, the person just gets fatter and fatter, day by day, because their insulin level prevents them from using body fat for energy.

You see how what seems like overeating or being lazy can come *after* the weight gain, because the weight gain was due to high levels of insulin. And the high levels of insulin can come from eating a normal number of calories on a high carb diet.

If the Government Recommendation Can Lead to Obesity, Why Is It Still Recommended?

I don't think there was a conspiracy to get Americans to be overweight or obese or to start a Type 2 diabetes epidemic. I believe the dietary guidelines offered by the government haven't changed for several reasons related to simple human nature:

1. <u>The belief that obesity is an issue of willpower and drive</u>: If you believe people get fat because they eat too much and don't exercise enough, there is no reason to think the guidelines are wrong—you just assume people are overeating and under exercising. Under this assumption the solution is "eat less" and "get moving" campaigns—like you see these days. When they don't work, you blame the dieter for not sticking to it.

2. <u>Cognitive dissonance</u>: No one involved with the guidelines wants to admit the government has given bad advice that has led to a lot of unnecessary sickness and death. I think the people who came up with the guidelines had good intentions; they just didn't test the guidelines before issuing them, and it turned out that they were wrong. Admitting the guidelines were wrong could lead to millions of people looking for compensation for this bad advice that has led to their ill-health and/or the death of loved ones.

3. <u>Pressure from the food industry to avoid the topic</u>: The US food industry has spent the last several decades developing low-fat foods. If the dietary guidelines were to change so dramatically, the industry could lose billions of dollars while they develop new, high fat foods.

4. <u>Pressure from the pharmaceutical industry to avoid the topic</u>: The Pharmaceutical industry also makes billions of dollars off of the results of the current US dietary guidelines. Sales of insulin and other drugs prescribed to diabetics and those determined to have "pre-diabetes" would be at risk if the guidelines were to change to a low-carb/high-fat diet. As is discussed in Appendix FAT, a low-carb diet also improves one's cholesterol and triglyceride levels—making a host of other drugs, like statins, unnecessary.

In any event, the low-fat diet recommendation is still the official stance of the US government. Even the Centers for Disease Control (CDC), in their suggested diet for diabetics, recommend a low-fat diet. I can only imagine that the CDC has to follow the USDA recommendation so as not to offer a governmental conflict. But knowing what you know now, you can see the absurdity of suggesting to people who can't properly metabolize glucose in the blood to eat 65% of their calories as carbohydrates, and then inject themselves with insulin to rid the blood of the glucose they take into their body each day.

The fields of Medicine and Nutrition are in a difficult position when it comes to the healthy proportions of the three macronutrients:

- They reject the notion of a high-protein diet because of a belief that too much protein can lead to kidney problems—so they limit protein to 20% of calories, which is about all that most people want to eat at any one time anyway.
- They have endorsed the importance of a <u>low-fat</u> diet to combat heart disease—so no more than 25% of calories from fat.
- The first two points determine that 55% of calories have to come from carbohydrates (100% - 20% - 25% = 55%).

But we know that eating that many carbs can cause insulin resistance, obesity and Type 2 diabetes. Type 2 diabetes, in turn, can lead to heart disease, which is what the low-fat diet was supposed to protect us from. Said another way: ***To fight heart disease, the fields of Medicine and Nutrition, along with the US government, recommend a diet that, in the end, leads to heart disease.*** I told you some of the facts would be hard to believe.

In my view, the tragedy of this situation is that if these groups would just look at the evidence, they would see that:
- High amounts of protein have been shown to actually improve kidney function rather than hurt it. Stuart Phillips, a professor of kinesiology at McMaster University, who oversaw a re-analysis of the results of 28 research studies said "It's a concept that's been around for at least 50 years and you hear it all the time: higher protein diets cause kidney disease. The fact is, however, that there's just no evidence to support this hypothesis; in fact, the evidence shows the contrary is true: higher protein [in the diet] increases, not decreases, kidney function."[6]
- A low-fat diet *doesn't* protect against the heart disease risk factors it was once thought to protect us from—and there is evidence that a **high-fat** diet is actually good for the body and the heart in particular (see Appendix FAT).
- Historically, obesity and Type 2 diabetes were treated successfully with a low-carb diet.
- Since Type 2 diabetes can lead to heart disease, a low-carb/high-fat diet protects us from a major cause of heart disease. (The other major cause is smoking.)

How this evidence could point to anything but a low-carb/high-fat diet as being the diet to protect us from heart disease (and a long list of other illnesses) is completely beyond me.

How to Get (and Stay) Lean

Why the Advice the Doctor Gives You to Lose Weight Typically Doesn't Work

The "eat less/move more" approach has been prescribed for weight loss for decades. Typically, it works well for the first few weeks. You cut back on the food you eat and go to the gym or walk more—and you start to lose weight. Then after a few weeks your weight loss slows down, and then it stalls. Soon after, even though you are watching what you eat and exercising, you start gaining weight! Then, if you are like me, you give up, only to start the same process after a year or so. And, of course, everyone blames you for not having the willpower to stick to the plan.

This cycle happens to almost everyone who tries it. Why? The "eat less/move more" approach to weight loss is based on the belief that the amount of energy going into your body (the amount of food you eat) and the amount of energy your body uses, are independent of each other—that is, it is assumed that you can lower the amount of energy going into the body without impacting the amount of energy your body uses.

This belief is just wrong[18].

Our bodies regulate our weight like they regulate our temperature. If we get too hot, we sweat to cool ourselves down; when we are too cold, we shiver to warm up. And we do these things automatically—they are really beyond our conscious control. For example, if we are out on a hot, humid day, we can't keep ourselves from sweating.

A similar thing happens with your weight—especially when you primarily metabolize (burn) carbs for energy. First, I'll describe how the weight regulation system works. Then I'll explain what happens when the system is running primarily on glucose (the sugar from carbs).

The full explanation of the regulatory system for weight is much too complex for this book. If you are interested in the full story, check out "The Physiology of Body Weight Regulation"[12]. Our understanding of the full story is still being researched—more is learned each year as more research is done. The article I just referenced strays a bit from what I've presented here, but their discussion of some of the hormonal and enzyme regulators of weight are on target. And while it is, to a large extent, an overview, the article contains further references if you want to go even deeper.

The simplified weight-regulation system looks like this:

Your body needs a certain amount of energy to run on each day to live. We talk about this amount of energy in terms of calories (it's actually kilocalories, but we just call it calories). You can look online for "Basal Metabolic Rate" charts that show how many calories, on average, a man or a woman needs, per day, to function given their height and weight. For me, it's 2165. That means that if my insulin levels and response to food are normal, and I eat 2165 calories a day, my weight will stay stable. How does that work since I don't know, day-to-day, how many calories I'm eating **or** using!

Your body keeps track of your energy. Not in terms of calories—there is no calorie counter in your brain. But if you are "insulin-normal" (that is, if your insulin levels and response are normal, and all the other hormones that regulate weight are normal) your brain understands your current energy balance. But it's not something you are directly conscious of—it's one of those systems that work in the background, like temperature control[13][14].

If the weight-control system in my body is working correctly, and I eat 2300 calories instead of 2165, my body would get me to move more than usual—I might get fidgety or feel like going for a long walk[15]. Or I might just get a little warmer if I resist moving more since we burn calories to create body heat. I'm not consciously aware that my body is trying to work off those extra calories, but that's what it's doing. The system wants to maintain an energy balance.

If I move too little (if I use fewer than 2165 calories), my body will send me signals that I don't need to eat so much—I might skip a meal "because I just don't feel hungry" or I will get full sooner than usual, before finishing my meal—or I'll decide to just eat a small meal. Again, the system wants to maintain an energy balance.

Here is the Reason the Eat Less/Move More Diets DON'T Typically Work Long-Term[16]:

Let's say that for my attempt to lose weight, I cut back to 1865 calories a day—a 300 calorie per day "deficit," as they say in the diet industry. Does my body notice this? You bet it does! If I eat 1865 calories instead of 2165, I'll get hungrier and want to eat more—my body wants me to hit that 2165 calorie energy balance target. My conscious brain knows I want to lose weight, but the subconscious brain doesn't know—it's an automatic system.

Okay, but I do know I want to lose weight, so I can decide to live with the hunger. If I do that, my body responds by lowering my Basal Metabolism—that is, it slows me down, so I don't use up as much energy. It can take a few weeks for this to happen. But it will happen.   If I eat 1865 calories a day, eventually, by body will slow me down so I only use 1865 calories a day. I'll find myself driving to the store instead of walking. I'll sit in front of the TV instead of going for that bike ride. It's an automatic system that tries to balance the energy used based on the energy coming in.
And "moving more" makes the calorie deficit worse! If I'm eating 1865 calories and burning an extra 300 at the gym, I have a 600 calorie per day deficit. After a month or so, what had been good weight loss progress will start to slow down—because my body is trying to balance the energy going out to what's coming in.

Worse yet, my body will remember I used to weigh more[17]. To help me gain back the weight I lost, it lowers my basal metabolism so much that even at a 600-calorie deficit from the 2165 I used to eat, I gain weight. So, while I'm eating 1865 and exercising to an effective rate of 1565 calories per day (a 600-calorie deficit from my original 2165), my body will slow down to maybe 1365—so I start gaining weight. I can try to fight this process and exercise even more and eat even less, but in the end I'll be so hungry and tired all the time I'll end up eating more and exercising less, and I'll gain all the weight back—just like my body wants. You can see why Dr. Jason Fung, in his book "The Obesity Code," says "the caloric-reduction theory of obesity was as useful as a half-built bridge."[19]

Now, in a body that is insulin resistant (like mine and many overweight or obese people) the problem is amplified. It's amplified because we don't have access to the stored energy from fat, or from all the food we eat after we eat it, because insulin stops the usage of body fat for fuel and puts a lot of the excess potential energy from the food we eat into our fat cells (which stays there because our insulin levels are always high enough to halt the production of the fat-burning hormone, glucagon).

So, if the chart says I should eat 2165 calories a day and I measure and eat 2165 calories exactly, but my resting insulin level is high, my body will see that as a deficit—because not all 2165 calories will be available to me. Because of the high insulin levels in my blood, some of the energy from those calories will be stored and trapped in my fat cells. As I mentioned earlier in the book, this is why overweight/obese people are always hungry and/or don't move a lot. It's because to their body, they are restricting the calories available when they eat the "recommended" number of calories—so their weight-control system makes them want to eat more calories and/or use less energy.

The overweight person is responding to the same signals the lean person is. When a lean person's body recognizes a deficit in calories, it makes the lean person hungry and gets them thinking about food. The same thing happens with overweight and obese people. To the outside world it LOOKS like the overweight person is overeating when they have their second Big Mac. But the part of the obese person's subconscious energy-balance system that "sees" how much energy is available to them doesn't see all of the first Big Mac—so it sends signals to eat more. And these signals are no more under the control of the overweight person than anyone's ability to not sweat on a hot, humid day.

The simple solution

Research has shown that simply eating a low-carb/high-fat diet can correct, and reverse, weight gain and diseases related to high blood sugar like obesity and Type 2 diabetes. You've seen the evidence. If you want to **stop storing** too much fat and, instead, **burn** fat for fuel, switching to a low-carb/high-fat diet is your best bet to accomplish this goal.

Does this make sense given what we've discussed in this book so far? Absolutely!

Q: What happens when we eat a low-carb diet?
A: Insulin goes down. And when insulin goes down, glucagon can do its job. And when glucagon does its job, we start burning fat—both the fat we eat, and the fat stored in our body.

Q: But what about the 5 grams of glucose we need in our blood?
A: Our liver can create all the glucose we need out of stored body fat.

Q: But what happens when we run out of fat to burn or make glucose out of?
A: You won't run out of fat. Even top athletes have body fat—much less than the rest of us, but probably about 10% of their body weight is fat. The body regulates fat storage and will ensure you keep enough for daily use.

An interesting thing about eating more fat in the diet is you tend to actually feel full—instead of just realizing you've eaten a lot of food and should probably stop. Feeling full leads you to eat less than you would on a high carbohydrate diet—highly processed carbs can bypass the signaling that you are full. So, you eat great-tasting food until you get full and lose or maintain your weight at the same time.

I was initially very skeptical about this approach. While it made sense according to the science of how our bodies react to food, it just seemed too simple to be true. But I tried it anyway! I lowered my carbs to as little as 20 grams a day and it helped me lose over 175 pounds—and keep it off. And aside from giving up a lot of carbs (which can be delicious as well as addicting!) the weight loss and weight maintenance has been effortless.

Will a low-carb/high-fat diet lead everyone to get and/or stay lean? It's hard to say. In my opinion, if you are overweight and eat a low-carb/high-fat diet and gain weight or fail to lose weight after a month or two, you have an unusual (probably hormonal) issue going on and should see a specialist. Of course, if you have gotten lean and are staying lean, that's not a problem. The low-carb/high-fat diet won't promote fat loss forever—your body will regulate itself and adjust to what you eat to maintain your weight. You just need to listen to the signals your body sends you—eat when you are hungry; stop eating when you are full.

Keep in mind, also, that while our bodies are *like* a machine, they aren't machines. With a machine, reactions to changes are typically quick and very predictable: If you switch a flex-fuel engine from gasoline to E85, the power output will change immediately and in a predictable way. But that's not how our bodies respond to changes.

A change in diet might spark immediate weight loss for some. Mine took about a week—quick, but not immediate. Some might take a few weeks to notice a change. Also, sticking to the diet, once weight loss kicks in, doesn't guarantee a consistent amount of weight loss week to week. Our bodies sense and react, re-sense and re-react.

Remember, weight control is a process. We can't control how the process works. But we **can** control when to start and stop the process (when we eat and the time we leave between meals) and what gets processed (the food we eat). Both of these things have a huge impact on our weight.

This simple low-carb/high-fat (LCFH) approach works within the process your body is going to use—the process your body has to use. That's the beauty of the approach! You can't download a new metabolic process into your body—you have to work within the rules of your body. Your body reacts to reduced calorie intake by making you hungry—and if you resist eating, it's going to slow down your metabolism to match the calories you are eating or even to the point where you start gaining weight with the reduced number of calories you do eat. That's why the "eat less/move more" advice almost never works in the long-term: It's fighting against how your body works.

The simple, LCHF approach, works because it is in line with how your body has to process food. You just need to adapt what and when you eat to work with the process your body needs to follow. Eat very few carbs and your body will switch over to burning fat for fuel. It's that simple.

Your body has to pump a lot of insulin into your blood if you eat a lot of carbohydrates. If you are eating a low-carb diet, the extra fat you end up eating (I focus on eating saturated fat (mostly from animal sources) or monounsaturated fat (like from cold-pressed, extra virgin olive oil)) will likely improve your health. Controlled research studies of low-carb/high-fat diets (again, see Appendix FAT) among adults show that compared to the USDA-recommended low-fat diet, <u>a low-carb/high-fat diet improves many of the things doctors suggest are signs of a heart attack just waiting to happen</u>: Higher HDL cholesterol numbers, lower amounts of fat in the blood (serum triglycerides), weight loss, better glucose control and lower blood pressure. And there are many practicing doctors working with sufferers of Type 2 diabetes who have seen patients reduce the amount of insulin they need to inject—or even the need for injected insulin at all—just from changing to a low-carb/high-fat diet!

How I Approached Eating A Low-Carb/High-Fat Diet

Rather than counting how many calories I eat each day, I keep track of how many grams of carbohydrates I eat. I count *grams* of carbs because the nutrition labels on food (and in nutrition apps) show the amounts of macronutrients in grams. The following details how I moved to and continue to eat a low-carb/high-fat diet: how I count my daily grams of carbs using nutrition labels and a free carb-tracking app (at least it was free as of the writing of this book; if the one suggested here has started charging, find another free one!):

First, I used one of those online calorie calculators to determine how many calories I should be eating per day. For me it was 2,165 calories (now it's fewer because I've lost weight and need less energy to move around). I don't count calories per day—but you need a starting point for the next step.

Next, I determined how many calories to get from carbs—I wanted my net carbs (grams of carbohydrates minus grams of fiber) to be a maximum of 5% of my calories. Five percent of 2,165 is 108 calories. In the European Union the grams of carbohydrate shown are net carbs.

At 4 calories per gram, 108 calories equates to 27 grams of net carbs (108 calories ÷ 4 calories/gram = 27 grams). I use 20 grams as my target—that way if I go a little over, I still keep it under 27 grams.

When I started this low-carb/high-fat approach to eating I tracked all 3 macronutrients—but now I just count my carbs and consciously try to add fat to my meal. Then I just eat until I'm full. If you have been overweight for a long time, like I was, feeling the sense of being full, and using it as a cue to stop eating, is something you might need to relearn. I would plan out and count my carbs (using the app found at www.cronometer.com), but then just eat until I was full; not bursting, just full. What works for you might be different. In my opinion, the specific route you take to low-carb/high-fat is less important than the final destination!

Tracking Carbs

To track your carbs (and protein and fat), you need to look at food labels. The "Cronometer" tracker app has a nice feature where you can scan the barcode of a food package and it downloads the macros for you. You just enter the amount (in grams, ounces, or servings) you eat, and your macros are tracked. You can also enter unprocessed foods like beef, chicken, eggs, fruits and vegetables. This particular app will give you a running total of your 3 macronutrients for the day. I'm not saying the app I use is the best—I didn't really look at too many. I came upon this one and liked it, so I use it. So, check out a few until you find one you like.

Even if you use an app to track, it's helpful to look at nutrition labels on processed food if for no other reason than to become aware of just how much sugar is used in processed food! Here is an example nutrition label for a brand of pretzels:

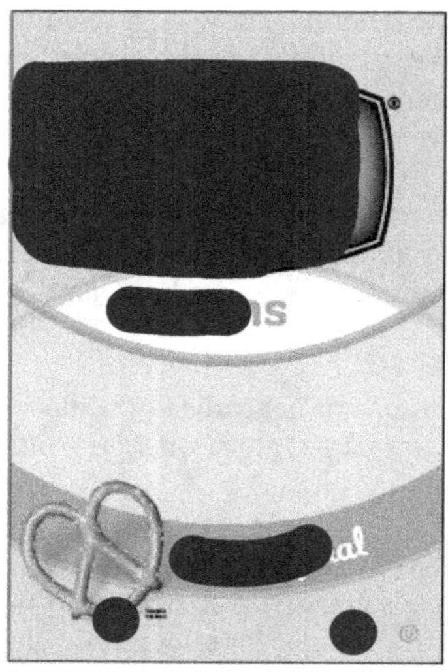

Nutrition Facts

Serving Size 1 oz (28g/About 9 pretzels)

Amount Per Serving	
Calories 110	Calories from Fat 10

	% Daily Value*
Total Fat 1g	**2%**
Saturated Fat 0g	**0%**
Trans Fat 0g	
Cholesterol 0mg	**0%**
Sodium 490mg	**20%**
Total Carbohydrate 23g	**8%**
Dietary Fiber 1g	**4%**
Sugars less than 1g	
Protein 2g	

Vitamin A 0%	•	Vitamin C 0%
Calcium 0%	•	Iron 8%
Thiamin 8%	•	Riboflavin 4%
Niacin 6%	•	Phosphorus 2%

* Percent Daily Values are based on a 2,000 calorie diet. Your daily values may be higher or lower depending on your calorie needs:

	Calories:	2,000	2,500
Total Fat	Less than	65g	80g
Sat Fat	Less than	20g	25g
Cholesterol	Less than	300mg	300mg
Sodium	Less than	2,400mg	2,400mg
Total Carbohydrate		300g	375g
Dietary Fiber		25g	30g

Calories per gram:
Fat 9 • Carbohydrate 4 • Protein 4

Ingredients: Enriched Flour (Wheat Flour, Niacin, Reduced Iron, Thiamin Mononitrate, Riboflavin, Folic Acid), Salt, Corn Syrup, Corn Oil, Malt Extract, Yeast, and Ammonium Bicarbonate.
CONTAINS A WHEAT INGREDIENT.

The first thing to notice is the serving size: 1 ounce (28 grams) or about 9 pretzels. 28 grams is the actual weight of the pretzels (not carbohydrates in the pretzels) that the nutrient data are based on. If you have 56 grams, or 18 pretzels, you will need to double the nutrient grams.

From there, all you really need to focus on is **Total Carbohydrates and Dietary Fiber**. Note that the number of grams of carbohydrates in the 28 grams of pretzels is 23 grams; with 1 gram of dietary fiber. The net carbs for 28 grams of these pretzels is 22 (23 − 1 = 22).

These 28 grams of pretzels account for nearly all of the grams of net carbs of my limit (27 grams) and more than all I aim for each day (20 grams).

Let that sink in. You will likely need to get your carbs down to the equivalent of 9 pretzels a day if you go as low-carb as I did! I'm not saying you need to go this low. I did because it helped me drop weight quickly—but it is a bit of a challenge at first.

If you are like me, you'll go through withdrawal symptoms. I looked at not eating carbs as a kind of medicine—a medicine you take by not taking it. If a doctor told me I needed to take bad-tasting medicine to treat a condition I had, I'd do it. Most of us would. Well, NOT EATING a lot of carbs is the medicine I need to take because I produce too much insulin when I eat a lot of carbs—and then I get fat. I looked at the withdrawal symptoms (discussed later) as being worth it. And they only lasted a week or so.

Side Note: There is also something called the "Glycemic Index" (GI) of foods[30]. The GI is a way of looking at how carbs from a specific food impact our insulin level relative to the impact pure glucose has. The GI of pure glucose is 100. Everything else has an index lower than 100. For example, the GI for white bread is 71; the GI for grapefruit is 25.

Some people will factor down their grams of carbs by the GI. For example, half of a grapefruit has about 11 grams of net carbohydrates. Someone using the GI would say that half a grapefruit would have only 2.75 grams of carbs: 11 grams x (GI/100) which works out to 11 grams x .25 = 2.75. As you can see, using this approach lets you eat more carbs and stay under your limit. Personally, this is just too complicated—I don't want to pull out my calculator every time I eat to factor down the carbs; I just count the net carbs. I am trying to learn which carbs have a lower GI because for me, the fewer effective carbs the better.

Also, some point out how the GI can be misleading to the extent the food you eat contains fructose. Pure fructose has a GI of 0 (zero) because it contains no glucose. But fructose can have a devastating effect on your fat storage. For this reason alone, some consider the GI to be worse than useless.

As you can see, you do need to nearly give up a lot of foods. But there are a lot of delicious foods you **can** eat as well (notice that bacon has zero carbs!):

Food	Grams of Total Carbohydrates per 100 grams of food (unless noted otherwise)	Grams Net Carbs	% of My Goal Limit of 20 grams/day
White Bread	15 (per slice)	13	65%
Mac & Cheese	50 in 1 serving (1/3 of the box)	49	245%
Potatoes	26 each	24	120%
Rice	28	27	135%
Peas	80	64	320%
Green Beans	7	5	25%
Carrots	10	7	35%
Celery Sticks	3	1	5%
Spinach	4	2	10%
Broccoli	6	3	15%
Romaine Lettuce	3	2	10%
Iceberg Lettuce	3	2	10%
Apples	14	12	60%
Bananas	23	20	100%
Grapes	18	15	75%
Oranges	13	10	50%
Pears	16	13	65%
Strawberries	7	5	25%
Any kind of Milk	11 (in 8 ounces)	11	55%
Corn Flakes	24 (in 1 ounce/28 grams/1 serving)	23	115%
Frosted Flakes	26 (in 1 ounce/28 grams/1 serving)	26	130%
Bacon	0	0	0%
NY strip steak	0	0	0%
Chicken breast	0	0	0%
Pork chops	0	0	0%
Pork shoulder	0	0	0%
Salmon	0	0	0%
Trout	0	0	0%

Tuna (canned)	0	0	0%
Hamburger (80% lean)	0	0	0%
Avocado	9	2	0%

I've highlighted anything particularly low in carbs in **bold** and anything particularly high in carbs in *italics*. As you can see, using Total Carbs is about the same as using Net Carbs for many foods.

There are some surprising numbers in the table! With that in mind, I urge you to look at the carb content of foods as you transition away from carbs.

That said, just for the sake of comparison, to get 9 pretzel's worth of net carbs (22) from vegetables, you'd need to eat 730 grams (over 1.5 pounds) of broccoli, or 1.1 kilo (almost 2.5 pounds) of lettuce! You could even have about a half-pound of grapes or oranges and get the same net carbs as found in 1 ounce of pretzels.

If you are used to the recommended high carb diet, going low-carb will be a jolt to your system. Sugar is as addictive as a drug—so withdrawal can be at best, annoying! I reduced my carbs from USDA recommended to 20 grams a day in steps. I didn't stay on any one step for very long, but I didn't make any big jumps, either. I cut out types of food as opposed to tracking my declining carb eating. (I started my low-carb journey before knowing all the information in this book!) For example, I stopped eating pretzels and pasta first. Then I stopped eating cereal and bananas for breakfast. I found this relatively easy because I just stopped buying these foods. If the foods weren't in the house, I couldn't eat them!

I also cut out snacks and sweetened soft drinks. I switched to drinking sparkling water. The carbs I eat now come mostly from vegetables and things otherwise high in fat like avocados and nuts. That said, we still need to live life! I live in Italy now, so I still have a pizza from time to time. And when at a social gathering, carbs usually pop up. So, there are days where I'll go way over my 20 grams a day limit. Sometimes, the next day, I'll try to stick to 10 grams of carbs; other times I just get back to 20 grams. My point is, I aim for my 20 grams a day—but I don't obsess over it if I go over once in a while. The important thing is to make "once in a while" REALLY once in a while.

Eating a lot of carbs while you transition to being primarily a "fat burner" (fat adapted) can lead to feeling sort of hung-over the next morning. Again, sugar/glucose is like a drug. Transitioning is like going through withdrawal. Once you are fat adapted, occasional higher-carb days can be helpful in teaching your body to switch back to burning fat without the hangover symptoms. Like I said earlier, your body is NOT a machine. It has to get used to changes.

Once you are fat adapted and used to eating a low-carb diet, you won't need to think too much about it. It will just be how you eat. For me, the biggest challenge is going out to eat with friends. If the group orders appetizers that are carb heavy, I'll either order something extra that is more protein/fat oriented or just nibble at the shared appetizers. My friends and family know I eat low-carb. After seeing the results of my weight loss, no one puts up a fuss about it.

Notes on transitioning from being a carb-burner to being a fat-burner:

IF YOU ARE ON MEDICATION, discuss your low-carb/high-fat plans with your doctor as with your weight loss, your dosage of medication might need to change.

Withdrawal symptoms while transitioning can include:
- Fatigue
- Nausea
- Light-headedness
- Cravings

Use your judgment on how quickly to lower your carb intake. Go as slow as you need to. If you can tough it out, the rewards can be great!

When you start primarily burning fat, you might notice your breath has a different smell. You might also notice you have more energy—because your body realizes it has a vast store of energy in and around your body, so it doesn't hold you back. You might also notice you don't get hungry as often as you did when you were a carb-burner. That was a real surprise for me. I just stopped having the hunger pangs I used to get around mealtime. I still enjoy eating, it's just that the "I'm starving" feeling doesn't hit me very often.

The hardest thing about a low-carb/high-fat diet is preparing and eating the high fat food. We live in a culture that has wrongly blamed dietary fat for all sorts of diseases when the real culprits are sugar, refined carbohydrates and bad oils (see Appendix ONE MAN'S EGO and Appendix FAT for more details).

For more details on why a low-carb/high-fat diet works and why the eat less/move more approach typically fails, read Appendix ADULTS ONLY.

A HEALTHY DIET

To summarize, a lot of us get fat from eating too many carbohydrates—both in the form of sugar as well as the refined carbohydrates found is highly-processed food products. We can get fat even eating the recommended number of calories if we eat the amount of carbs the government guidelines tell us. In fact, let's look at the graph of levels of adult obesity and being overweight. This time I've added when the USDA food guidelines were introduced.

% of US Adults, 20 – 74, Classified as Obese or Extremely Obese[1]

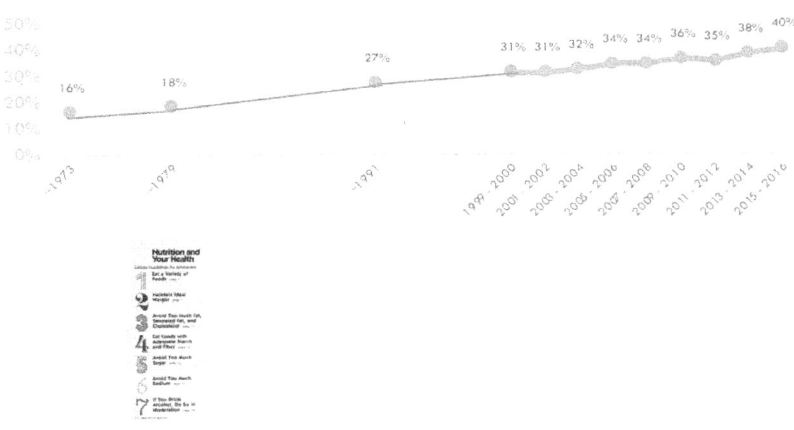

How Much of Each Macronutrient Do We Need?

It's tempting to call the question of what's the right balance of macronutrients "the age-old question." But it's really a rather recent question in the context of human history. For hundreds of thousands of years, our ancient ancestors, like animal species around the world that self-feed, ate the foods that kept them healthy and lean.

So, what happened to change this? I, and many in the field of nutrition, think it had to do with changes in our diet—changes in the types and amounts of food we ate. Before beginning the story behind the drastic change in our diet, I want to be clear that **I DO NOT** think there was some sort of conspiracy to cause an obesity epidemic. I just think several events and people came together in a way that was unfortunate for many, including myself.

In his book "The Case Against Sugar," Gary Taubes, a brilliant investigative journalist focusing on science issues, points to sugar as a major factor in the rise of diabetes. In his book, which I highly recommend, Gary lays out a very detailed history of the sugar industry and what happened in the US when a new method for producing sugar was produced that drastically reduced the cost of sugar. With the low cost, sugar use increased.

It's difficult to get medical statistics from the 1800s, but it seems diabetes was an extremely rare disease. As recently as 1958, the CDC reports, only 1% of the US population had been diagnosed with diabetes. As of 2015, that number has risen to 9.4% of Americans. And in a recent CDC report[10] from 2017, it is estimated that an additional 26% are likely to have diabetes within the next 5 years. That would bring the US rate of diabetes up to 35% by 2022!

It would seem that sugar played a role in the increase in obesity (which often is a sign of diabetes in the making). Once sugar became cheap, it showed up in all sorts of foods and gave birth to the candy and soft drink industries. Sugar was moving from being a rare treat to a dietary staple.

In the 1950s, then-president Eisenhower had a heart attack. Heart disease had been rising steadily since after World War 1 (American soldiers were given cigarettes as part of their rations and continued to smoke when they returned—starting a fad that took off; it's interesting to note that by that time, cigarettes were treated with sugar to make the smoke more tolerable!). Eisenhower's heart attack got the country to focus on heart disease. A physiologist at the University of Minnesota, Ancel Keys, had a hypothesis. Ancel Keys is the man who developed the food packages (the K-Rations) soldiers were issued in World War 2—so he had a relatively high profile, especially with Eisenhower, a five-star general during the war.

Keys believed that eating fat is what caused heart attacks. Apparently, Eisenhower was fond of sausage and eggs for breakfast, and Keys pointed to the excess fat in the president's diet as the culprit. Keys either didn't realize, or chose to ignore, the fact that Eisenhower was also a chain-smoker.

Keys' theory was that a diet <u>low in fat</u> would cure the nation of its epidemic of heart disease. He even showed some data, collected from countries around the world, that supported his hypothesis that there was a link between fat in the diet and death from heart disease. The data he showed are presented in Appendix ONE MAN'S EGO. For now, it's enough to say his presentation of the data was fraudulent. Out of the 22 countries he collected data from, he only showed the 6 data points that fit his theory. This wasn't science. In science, your theory should arise from the data. Keys did it backwards—he had a theory and cherry-picked the data that supported his idea.

To summarize what is in the appendix, Keys eventually got the American Heart Association to back the low-fat diet—and a new epidemic was born (oh, and by the way, the move to a low-fat diet has not improved the rate of heart disease—moving away from smoking has).

⌕ Key Points to Remember:
- The rates of diabetes (a frequent condition that develops with obesity) went up after the introduction of cheap sugar in the US.
- A low-fat diet recommendation was backed by the American Heart Association. The low-fat diet was the idea of Ancel Keys.
- Keys thought dietary fat caused heart disease and showed a compelling chart to back up his idea.
- The chart was fraudulent as it didn't show all the data. Showing all the data didn't support Keys' idea.

In 1977, the US government published the Dietary Guidelines for Americans. This was the government's first attempt to guide our diet. On the left is the original 1977 version, and on the right, the second edition from 1985.

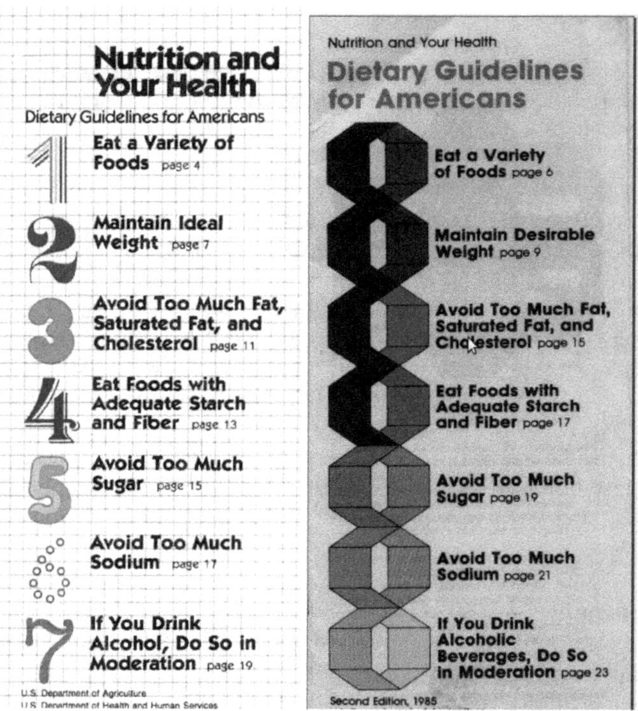

In eight years, the only changes were replacing the word ideal with desirable in point number 2, replacing the word alcohol with alcoholic beverages in point number 7 and getting rid of the numbers for each point!

Many of us are familiar with the food pyramid. This was produced by the US Department of Agriculture in 1992. It got regular updates and at one point was called My Pyramid. But the recommended servings of each food group remained basically the same over the years.

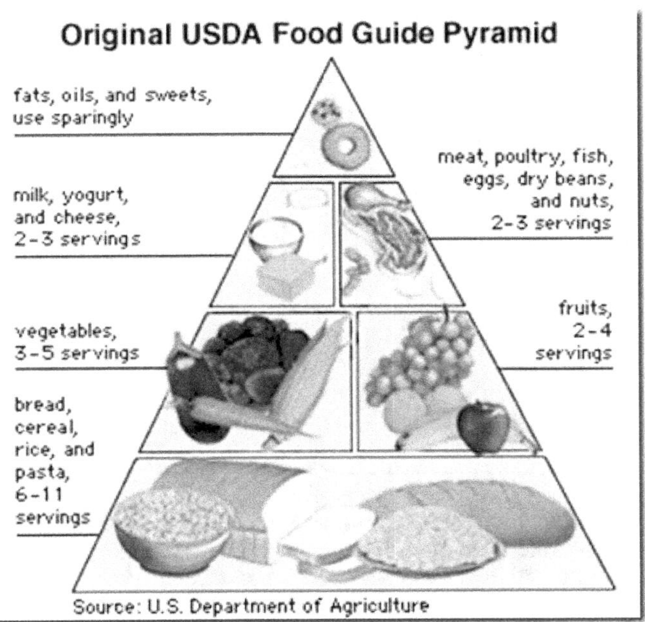

It's a bit odd that these food guidelines came from the Department of Agriculture. It would seem more appropriate coming from the Department of Health, Education, and Welfare, or what was left when Education because its own Cabinet-level department in 1979—the Department of Health and Human Services. The purpose of the US Department of Agriculture is to promote and regulate crops grown in the USA: Crops like grains, vegetables and fruit which make up the base of the pyramid—and our diet.

The original pyramid was based on the 1977/1985 guidelines and adapted by then Senator George McGovern, based on his own diet.

We now have the 2015 – 2020 guidelines. What was "the pyramid" is now "Choose My Plate." But nothing much beyond the name and the graphics has changed—grains, fruits and vegetables (agricultural products) still dominate the recommended diet.

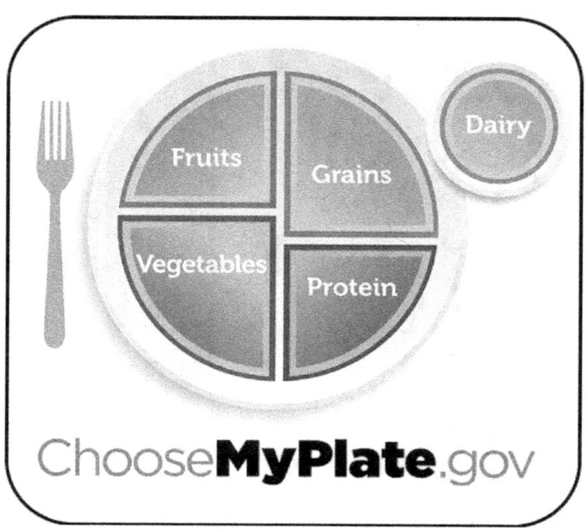

Well one thing that **has** changed is the serving suggestions for each food group. They've gotten more vague—like the original 1977 guidelines. Check out the web site: www.choosemyplate.gov/WhatIsMyPlate

If you do go through the actual 122 pages of guidelines, you will find, on page 97, that for ages 4 – 18, they still recommend: 10 – 30% of calories from protein, 25 – 35% from fat (with less than 10% coming from saturated fat) and 45 – 65% from carbohydrates (with less than 10% coming from added sugar). Babies—and it could be argued children in general—need more fat in their diet for brain and organ development. As such, the guidelines suggest a slightly higher percentage of fat for children aged 1 – 3: 5 – 20% protein, 30 – 40% fat (up 5 percentage points) and 45-65% carbohydrates. But the recommendations for 4 – 18 year-olds is almost the same as for those 19 and over: 10 – 35% protein, 20 – 35% fat and 45 – 65% carbs.[2]

🔎 **Key Points to Remember**:
- Despite its fraudulent start, the low-fat diet found its way into the American dietary guidelines.
- There have been several versions of these guidelines and they have taken many shapes—a list, a pyramid and a plate.
- Overall, since their beginning, the guidelines for Americans has stressed a **low-fat** diet.

If we take about the middle of each range of recommendations for macronutrients for adults we get:

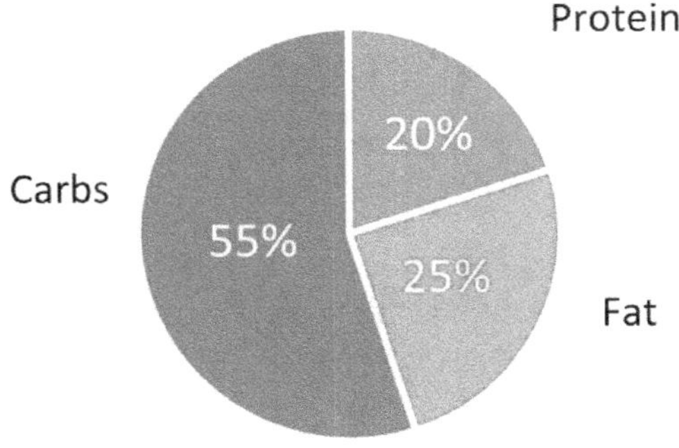

If we assume a diet of 2,000 calories, we need a diet that provides 1,100 calories per day from carbohydrates. At 4 calories per gram, that equals about 275 grams of carbs. That's the equivalent of over 1 pound of sugar per day (from the point of view of your blood). That's over 100 teaspoons of sugar per day (the image to the right is about 50 teaspoons-worth of sugar). Even if it was split equally over 3 meals and 2 snacks, it would still work out to over 20 teaspoons per eating occasion. That's a lot of sugar/glucose in the system, especially when you consider you have about 1 teaspoon in your blood at any given time.

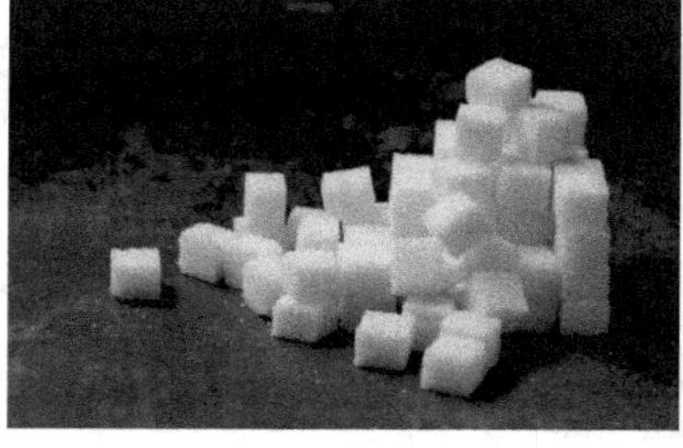

You might think there is no way you eat this much sugar. But it's not so difficult to do with the highly refined, ultra-processed foods on the market today.

For example:

Breakfast: 41 grams of carbs
A bowl of cheerios: 17 grams (net) carbs
1 banana: 24 grams (net) carbs
Coffee: 0 grams if taken without milk or sugar

Lunch: 155 grams of carbs
Amy's single serve pizza (which says it serves 3, so the nutrition info needs to be multiplied by three if you eat the whole thing—and why wouldn't you, it's a single-serve pizza!) gives you 90 grams (net) of carbs; add a 20 oz. Coke and you get another 65 grams of carbs. At least the bottle now says the 20 ounces is one serving.

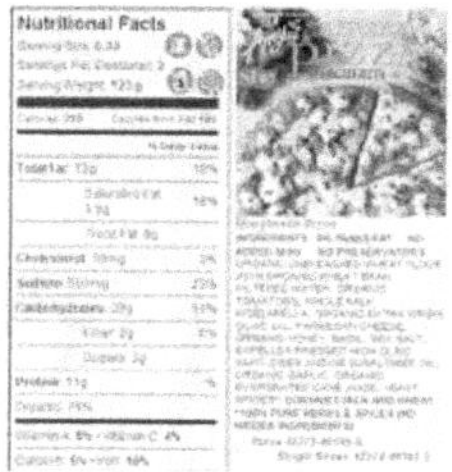

Snack: 16 grams of carbs
Low-fat blueberry yogurt: 16 grams of carbs

Dinner: 71 grams of carbs
Steak: 0 grams of carbs
Baked potato: 33 grams (net) of carbs
Asparagus: 3 grams (net) of carbs
Salad (romaine and tomatoes) with French dressing: 12 grams of carbs not counting the vegetables
Vanilla ice cream: 23 grams of carbs

Total for the day: 283 grams of carbs

Some people might be able to metabolize this much sugar without getting fat. Clearly, some of us cannot. Eating this many carbs, for many, leads to insulin resistance and a continuously growing amount of body fat, because glucagon never gets a chance to do its job.

Keep in mind that this can happen to people who are not overeating—this can happen eating the recommended number of total calories if the amount of carbs is too high for that individual. But when you are told to eat a low-fat diet for your health, you typically end up eating more carbs.

✎ Key Points to Remember
- Following the USDA recommended dietary guidelines leads you to eat the equivalent of over 1 pound of sugar per day.
- For many people, that translates to too much glucose for their system to handle and they get fat.
- Eating the recommended number of carbs on a low-fat diet (like the one recommended by the USDA guidelines) can lead a person to be obese.

But how much protein, fat and carbs do we need? Well, remember that there are no essential carbohydrates—if you don't eat any carbohydrates/sugar/glucose, your liver will produce 100% the glucose you need out of stored body fat.

Research that I've seen shows that there is a metabolic advantage—in terms of burning fat— to keeping carbohydrates to under 10% of total daily calories, but I shoot for 5%. I stick to the USDA recommendation on protein—between 20 and 30% of daily calories—and the rest of the diet as fat (65 – 70%).

I know it sound crazy and unhealthy! We've been told for decades that eating fat leads to heart and other health issues and/or makes us fat.

The reality, backed by research dating back to and before the big fat scare ushered in by Ancel Keys, is that dietary fat (the fat we eat) is not linked to health issues, and if eaten on a low-carb diet, does not lead to increased fat stores.

🔎 Key Points to Remember
- You don't need any carbs in your diet
- Research shows a metabolic advantage if carbs are kept to 10% or less of your daily calories.
- Eating a lot of fat, in the relative absence of carbohydrates promotes the burning of fat.

Summary

You learned a lot of information in a few dozen pages. It might be worth reading it again to help it sink in. To the extent the information was new to you, a second reading will help it become information you truly know; information that can guide your food decisions for the rest of your life.

You got a basic lesson in nutrition. You learned about the three macronutrients (protein, fat and carbohydrates) and how there are no essential carbs—while our body needs the basic building blocks of carbs (glucose), the liver can make all we need out of fat.

You got a basic lesson in metabolism. You learned how the body reacts to the different macronutrients. You saw how insulin is released into the blood to lower dangerous levels of blood sugar, and how insulin promotes the storage of fat and stops the body from burning fat. You also saw how when insulin levels drop, glucagon can do its job of promoting the burning of fat.

You saw that the information about nutrition and metabolism were used to come up with a healthy diet—a diet that our ancient ancestors likely ate, and a diet prescribed by doctors as far back as the 1800s. The idea of a low-carb/high-fat (LCHF) diet isn't new; it's not a "fad diet." It is a healthy diet—it can provide all the nutrients you need and helps with weight loss (if you are overweight) and weight maintenance (if you are lean).

You learned that many people get fat as a result of eating the USDA-recommended amount of carbohydrates each day. And you saw how when we see an overweight person "eating too much," it's likely that their body isn't able to use all the energy in the food they eat because their high insulin levels are storing some of that energy as fat before their body can use it to live on.

You learned how a low-carb/high-fat diet can lower resting insulin levels and allow glucagon to have a chance to burn the fat that insulin has stored. The LCHF diet allows the body to return to the rhythm of fat storage and fat burning we evolved to have.

You learned that highly processed foods contain a lot of sugar—because it sells more and increases the shelf-life of the product, and that even some fruits have been bred to contain more sugar for the same reasons. You learned how to look at nutrition labels to see just how many carbs are in the foods you eat.

You saw how I went from eating about 300 grams of carbs per day down to 20 grams per day. You saw how it can be hard to cut out so many carbs because sugar is addictive—you might go through a sort of carb withdrawal. But you also saw that I lost 175 pounds thanks to a low-carb diet!

You saw how if you are on medication, you should discuss your diet plans with your doctor because you might need to change your dosing as you lose weight.

As a final note, congratulations on the start of your journey to being lean for life!

PART 2: CHANGING YOUR APPROACH TOWARD FOOD

Steven asked me to write a section on food—including recipes—based on my experience as a chef. So here it is! I've added references and links to web articles and some research, but this section is not as science based as Part 1 of the book. So, take this information and my opinions with a grain of salt (which isn't as bad for you as we've been led to believe!).

Three of the issues related to changing our diet (and by "diet" I mean the range of foods we eat) are:
- Learning which foods to eat
- Learning which foods to avoid
- Our general attitude toward what is available.

The first two are fairly straightforward—they take some time to learn, but otherwise they aren't very difficult. The third one takes conscious effort and is critically important to how successful we will be with changing what and how we eat. Here, we have to decide if we will think about the foods we CAN'T EAT or the foods we CAN EAT.

When we concentrate on food we **can't eat**, we become myopic. We have tunnel vision. It's hard to think about, or even see, what we *can* eat when all we can think about are the things we can't have. This leads to cravings and generally makes life pretty miserable.

However, when we think about the bounty of foods we **can eat**, foods that fit into our new way of eating, we feel the freedom to pick and choose the foods we want. We don't feel deprived because we have many, many options to choose from. So, it is important, at the beginning, to develop a list of foods to buy and keep on hand—at the end of this section there is a list of the foods Steven and I have eaten along our paths to a LCHF diet that you can use for reference.

One of the nice things about restricting carbs is that you quickly stop craving them. If you eat more carbs, especially highly processed ones like breads and pasta, and you'll want more; cut back on them and the cravings disappear fairly quickly.

It really helps to just stop buying the foods you want to avoid. Don't have them in the house. If you don't have bread, pasta, rice, cookies, potatoes, etc. on hand, when it's time for dinner, you'll be eating meats, salads, and vegetables (assuming, of course, that those are your list and that's what you buy). Go so far as to avoid walking down the snack aisles in the grocery store. If you find yourself at the far end of the store, walk to the cashiers through the cleaning products aisle where you won't be tempted by tasty goodies.

While everything in this book, outside this section, is very current in nutritional science, and gives you a good understanding of where the food guidelines went wrong, and the horrible impact it's had, we have to keep in mind that nutrition is a relatively new science. We are just beginning to understand the intricate details of how things work, yet we are able to see the big impacts on weight, general health, metabolic diseases, across large populations and the correlations with diet tendencies.

In short: what we do know suggests that people are getting sick from eating diets high in carbs and highly processed foods. Such a diet follows when foods are made to be low in fat. Yes, some people, especially young people, seem to do just fine on such a diet. But are they really? Or are they just starting down the path that leads to poor health and they just aren't showing symptoms, yet?

Either way, the point is a bit moot. Something has brought you here, to read this book, something has gone wrong, and you'd like to fix it. And many diet-related issues can be fixed, simply by fixing your diet.

But keep this in mind: it is easy to fall into the trap that carbs are bad, so we should just eliminate carbs altogether. But I don't look at carbs in this way. I feel carbs have their place. It is just the overloading of carbs, especially highly processed ones, over a period of time, that causes the damage to our body.

Initially, to lose weight (and to reduce your insulin resistance, rid yourself of visceral fat, drop your triglycerides and raise your HDL, improve your blood pressure, stabilize coronary artery calcification, etc.,) you might want to go with a diet very low in carbs (like 20 grams/day, like Steven has been doing). Some people go all the way into a carnivore diet and they seem to do reasonably well on it. But, I have my reservations about going that stringent. My understanding, while meats and fats are certainly the most nutrient dense foods you can eat, the microbiome (gut health) also needs certain nutrients to survive, thrive, and support us.

Once you are lean, you can see where your carb limit can be and still keep your weight stable.

FOOD QUALITY

When you start learning about nutrition and food production you quickly start thinking about food quality. There are a lot of terms used on food packaging that try to convince you the food is of the highest quality: Organic, grass-fed, gluten-free, whole-grain, etc. But not all the terms mean what they suggest.

<u>Meat</u>: Let's look at the term "grass-fed." The term sounds like the grass-fed animals ate grass their entire life. But all that term means is that the animals ate grass <u>at some point in their life</u>. That time is usually at the beginning of their life (when they don't eat too much. Then, for the rest of their life they are fed grain—in the language of the beef industry, they were "finished" on a high grain diet. The same thing that makes us fat (overloading on carbs) makes cows fat as well. Fatter the cow is at auction, the higher price it gets, and the meat itself is fattier.

So, when you see "grass-fed" think "grass-fed, grain-finished."
"Grass-finished" means the cattle have eaten only grass their entire lives. The meat is leaner, has a better Omega-3 to Omega-6 ratio, and, some argue, has a wider variety of vitamins and minerals than grain-finished beef.

Ideally, we should eat grass-finished beef. Not only is it likely healthier for us, but it is also much better for the planet—that is, grass-feeding cattle is much friendlier to the environment than raising cattle on a feedlot.

Generally speaking, the above also applies to bison, goat, lamb and sheep – dairy cattle, and pastured pork.

For more information on grass-fed only standards, please go to[36]:

Grass-fed and grass-finished meats have been rising in popularity and every major grocery store I've been in, over the last few years, carry this product. However, supplies and types (cuts) are limited, and you will pay a premium price for them.

If you are concerned about hormones and antibiotics used on the animal (and you should be!), certified organic beef must come from cows that have never been treated with them; grass-finished beef is less likely to have been treated, but may have been; grain-finished, feedlot beef most certainly will have been treated with hormones and antibiotics.

This is a concern because when you eat the meat, you might be ingesting powerful hormones and antibiotics. I am not aware of any legitimate studies on this topic, and I imagine it would be somewhat difficult, and expensive, to do a proper study, but I play it safe and avoid "tainted" meat, if possible. I know someone who lives in Europe who worked in the US for about one year. She said her breasts grew a full cup size from the food (she didn't gain weight in general). She suspected the hormones in the meat as being the culprit as when she returned to Europe her breasts went back to their previous size.

For more on the topic of antibiotics in our food, go to[37]:
Antibiotics in Your Food: Should You be Concerned?

Regulations regarding the raising, and labeling, of chickens, in the United States, can also be misleading. It's easy to understand what "caged chickens" are, but what about "free-range?" Did these birds spend their life frolicking in the sunshine, pecking for worms, and nibbling on insects? Probably not. Free-range just means that they have access to the outside. So, how free was that chicken that you paid extra money for because it says free range on the package? It most likely came from a "factory farm" that housed 40,000 birds with one, possibly two, tiny doors that led outside. If it wanted to, it could go outside. Very few of them ever do make it to the outside, but that's all it takes to be able to call it a free-range chicken.

Pastured chickens, in theory, have actually been raised outside and some small studies suggest the meat is healthier. Like organic beef, organic chickens are not given antibiotics.

Fish, high in protein and Omega – 3 fatty acids, has been thought to be a superior food; especially albacore tuna, lake trout, mackerel, herring, and sardines. Two or more servings a week are considered beneficial by the American Heart Association.

But, in recent years, there have been fears raised about mercury in fish. The FDA (Food and Drug Administration – U.S.) believes up to 1 ppm (part per million) of methylmercury is safe and the average level of methylmercury in the U.S. seafood market, is .0.3 ppm. According to the FDA, "the top 10 seafood species—shrimp, pollock, salmon, cod, catfish, clams, flatfish, crabs, scallops and canned tuna—generally contain less than 0.2 ppm of methylmercury." They go on to recommend "only one 7-ounce helping per week of large fish, such as shark and swordfish. For seafood with lower levels of mercury, officials advise no more than 14 ounces per week." See **(Webmd)**[38] for more details.

PCB's[39], polychlorinated biphenyls, are highly toxic industrial compounds that were banned from manufacturing, in the U.S., in 1977. However, prior to that, starting in 1929, their use was widespread and even though they've been banned for over 40 years, they are still found in fish!

PCBs have been shown to cause a wide variety of health problems from causing cancer in animals as well as a number of other serious health issues in their immune system, reproductive system, nervous system, endocrine system, as well as other health effects. According to the EPA, there is evidence that PCBs have potential carcinogenic and non-carcinogenic effects on people, as well. **(EPA.gov)**

What about wild fish vs. farm-raised fish? Wild fish tend to be leaner, have a diverse diet, and higher levels of Omega-3 fatty acids than do farm-raised fish that are concentrated in tight environments and eat a restricted, limited diet. There are concerns that tilapia imported from China may be suspect as it is common, there, to feed tilapia animal feces. This may, or may not, introduce pathogens. Tilapia Fish: Benefits and Dangers[40]. **(Healthline.com)**

Wild-caught Salmon seems to be healthier, overall, than farmed salmon. In an attempt to reduce PCB's in farm raised salmon, they are fed fish pellets made with soy and grain. This results in salmon that has more fat (as we would expect!), but that fat is higher in Omega-6 fatty acids—which is not what you want if you are eating fish for their Omega-3 fatty acids.

So, there may be valid health reasons to choose wild-caught over farm raised fish; no matter what that fish may be. However, especially for some fish, like salmon and tilapia, you will pay a higher price for non-farm raised and you might not even be able to find it.

Now that we've briefly touched on wild versus farm raised fish, let's return to the overarching topic of the term "organic." While the term "organic" is legally defined, you should be skeptical, or at least become well informed, before spending extra money on something that says it's organic. It may or may not make a difference. It's true that there are certain processes that must be followed, and some practices are not allowed, like the use of sewer sludge for fertilizer. But certain synthetic chemicals can be used as long as they are approved by the National Organic Program of the U.S. Department of Agriculture. And we've already seen that the USDA isn't always up on the science related to agricultural products.

Here is a very good article on organic farming and its use of chemicals[41]: Mythbusting 101: Organic Farming > Conventional Agriculture.

"Natural" is a much vaguer term. The rules aren't as stringent and there is no certification process. It is only within the last five years or so that natural has meant anything at all. Prior to that natural could have, and did, mean anything the food manufacturer wanted it to mean.

For a better understanding of food labels, this article from LiveScience.com is a good source[42]: Food Labels: Definition of Natural & Organic.

You will probably be eating more cured meats, like ham, sausage, bacon, etc. if you have decided to follow a LCHF diet. Should you buy "uncured" meats because they aren't full of nitrates/nitrites? Personally, I save the dollar or two per package and buy the regular stuff. The uncured meat trend is just a marketing ploy. Both cured and uncured use nitrates/nitrites they are just derived from different sources. If you want to avoid nitrates, buy neither.

Here is an article from the Washington Post that addresses the issue[43]: The 'uncured' bacon illusion: It's actually cured, and it's not better for you.

At this point, you are probably wondering just how much you can trust the food manufacturers. I'd say they don't want to outright poison anyone, at least in a way that can get them into legal trouble or lead to a loss in sales or reputation. But it seems they put their interest in corporate profits over any interest in your health or well-being. Their job is to make money for shareholders, and they do that by providing you with food that you will buy regardless of its impact on your long-term health. If that means playing into food trends—no problem. Or if it means providing highly processed low-fat foods (filled with carbs to replace the fat), that's fine, too. And they can label it "heart healthy" if it is low in fat because the government still hasn't realized that it's the carbs—NOT THE FAT—in food that leads to heart disease.

As you've seen, much of what we thought we knew about food and nutrition was based on fraudulent research. But it was believed in so strongly it became the "facts" we were all told. If for no other reason but this, we are kind of on our own when it comes to nutrition and health. Therefore, it is our job to become somewhat knowledgeable about what we are eating and where it comes from.

<u>Fruits & Vegetables</u>: If you do all your produce shopping at a farmers' market, in season, chances are the vegetables were picked at their peak ripeness and nutritive value. They just haven't been sitting around long enough to degrade. The veggies you see at your local supermarket, for the most part, are a much different story. Vegetables in your local or chain supermarket might look nice, have good color, be firm to the touch. But they were picked before they were ripe and trucked into town—some from thousands of miles away. All they while they've been losing what nutritive value they started with.

Those firm, red tomatoes you buy in January—how healthy are they? About as healthy as they are flavorful! Yes, they are better than eating a donut, but that's a pretty low bar to set.

A better option, even during the summer (if you aren't buying local produce at a farmers' market), is frozen vegetables. They were picked at the optimal time, quickly blanched, then flash frozen. While there is some loss of nutritional value, it is nothing compared to the "fresh" stuff that has journeyed weeks and thousands of miles to get to you.

Frozen vegetables can also be easier to use, there's less waste, they are easier to portion out, and always available. I buy broccoli in five-pound freezer bags. I always have some on hand—makes my life easier! Tomatoes, sadly, don't freeze very well. The next best thing is to dry them out with some salt and crushed red pepper.

In addition to the above issues, there are questions concerning the declining nutritive value in the vegetables and fruits we purchase in the US[44]. Let's start with fruits: generally speaking, various fruits have been bred, over the last few hundred years, to become sweeter and sweeter. If you are following a LCHF diet, you probably aren't eating much, if any, fruit.

Vegetables are a different story, though. Because of mono-cropping, breeding plants to grow bigger, faster, and the use of pesticides, among other factors, vegetables have measurably less vitamins and minerals (such as protein, iron, riboflavin, calcium, and vitamin C to list just the most well-known) than those a few, short decades ago. That doesn't mean the vegetables are lacking in those vitamins and minerals, it just means there is less of them in the fruits and vegetables we eat today. Certainly, you should eat vegetables (that grow above the ground), but you should be aware of their nutritive value.

How do you know how much vitamins and minerals you are getting from the produce you buy? I don't think you can ever be certain, just assume you are getting some, and that what you are getting is still more nutritious than, say, a box of mac and cheese.

One alternative is to grow some of your own. Tending a garden is good for the body and the spirit. And you can buy seeds from the old-style vegetables we used to have, before the modern age of the food industry.

You should also have your doctor run a blood panel to see if you are deficient in the various vitamins and minerals. It's very unlikely, if you eat a well-rounded LCHF diet. But if you are in doubt, go ahead and have the blood work done.

Of course, figuring out the optimal amount of the various vitamins and minerals for you would be next to impossible—there are too many variables to take into account that impact what any one person needs. Age, ethnicity, general health, level of activity, along with many other factors, will change how much one person needs compared to any other person. So, the only way to really be confident that you are getting enough of these nutrients, is to eat as healthy a diet as you can and have the doctor run a test. Your body will run for years, and decades, with subpar nutrition and deficiencies, but once you get everything back in line, you'll feel, think, and do much better. (See Appendix VITAMINS & MINERALS for more details.)

OILS

This link to a Bon Appetit article[45] (<u>The Best Oils for Cooking, and Which to Avoid</u>)

is a worthwhile read—it's a primer on the oils commonly found in our markets and used in our foods. It is worth reading even if what I have to say might steer you away from using many of the oils listed. Canola, corn, soybean, peanut, sunflower, safflower, etc., (all vegetable/seed oils) are highly processed oils that rely on heat and petroleum solvents to extract the product. These oils are then deodorized, sometimes bleached, and sometimes hydrogenated to make them taste less noxious and be more shelf stable. Chemicals are also often used to make them the "right color".

From this point forward I will call them seed oils, as I don't want you to think I'm referring to healthy oils, like olive or avocado, that are pressed from the fruits but not subject to heating and chemical extraction.

<u>Why seed oils are bad for us</u>

Seed oils are a much-debated subject right now. The current guidelines state they are good for you and that you need to consume them daily. The problem is, by consuming seed oils, you are taking in too many omega-6 fatty acids.

Polyunsaturated fatty acids (PUFAs) contain omega-3 and omega-6 fatty acids. Both are considered "essential fatty acids" because our bodies need them, but our bodies can't make them out of other foods we eat. So, we have to eat foods containing omega-3 and omega-6 fatty acids. While we need both, we need to balance the amount of each we get—specifically, it's not good if we have more omega-6 relative to the amount of omega-3. Seed oils are chockful of omega-6 fatty acids. Overly high amounts of omega-6 have been linked to heart disease, diabetes, mitochondrial dysfunction, DNA damage, neurological disorders/amyloid plaques, macular degeneration, leptin resistance, and other health issues. That said, it is difficult to know the impact of seed oils on their own as they typically come hand-in-hand with a high-carb/highly processed diet. The good news is that if you switch to a LCHF diet, and use healthy oils, you will rid yourself of the risks from seed oils.

It appears that the damage from omega-6 fatty acids starts when our caloric intake is 4%, or more, of them. Seed oils, in animal tests, raised antioxidant enzyme activity whether the oil was unheated, singly heated, or repeatedly heated. They are bad for the body but get worse as you heat them[46].

Here is a well-written article from butterbeliever.com on vegetable/seed oils that is accurate and does a much better job of explaining it than I can[47]: <u>PUFA: What is it and Why Should it Be Avoided?</u>

<u>What About Olive Oil?</u> Now that we've decided to get rid of seed oils, and we are pretty sure that unheated olive oil is not only safe, but healthy, should we cook with olive oil? Polyunsaturated fats (seed oils) are sensitive to high heat (at the levels used for cooking). They go from bad to worse; they oxidize and form harmful compounds some of which are carcinogenic. Extra virgin olive oil is much more resistant to heat. To make it oxidize, and form bad compounds, it would need to be heated to an extreme temperature, for a such a long period of time, in conditions that you would never cook in. That's the good news.

The bad news is that heating olive oil will reduce some of its healthy compounds, but only when heated for longer periods (90 minutes). So, cooking with extra virgin olive oil is just fine. You may slightly degrade some of its benefits, but not by much and it's most likely worth it for the foods you want to eat. Olive oil isn't the only one you can cook with. Lard, schmaltz, beef tallow, clarified bacon grease, duck fat, and ghee, all have their uses, and each have their own flavor profile. One of the nice things about our modern society is being able to buy all of these items, usually at a reasonable price, locally or online. As with everything, it is worth doing some research to make sure you are getting a good quality product from a reputable company. Here is a good source for olive oil: <u>https://www.aboutoliveoil.org/certified-olive-oil-list</u>

"HEALTHY" WHOLE GRAINS

As you have seen, earlier in the book, most of us have grown up in a system that promotes the heavy use of grains. All the recommended lists, pyramids and plates issues by the USDA provide a clear message: Eat lots of carbs! Eat lots of grains and cereals!

<u>What are grains?</u> Generally speaking, grains (sometimes referred to as cereals) come from the grass family of plants. Grains are staple food throughout the world and are the dry, edible seeds of these grasses. Grains include: wheat, corn, oats, rice, wild rice, millet, barley, among others. Pseudo-grains, like quinoa and buckwheat, aren't actually grains, but they are prepared and consumed in a similar way.

Foods made from grains include breads, pasta, breakfast cereals, muesli, oatmeal, tortillas, as well as junk foods like pastries and cookies.

Some grains, like wheat, are very tough and almost impossible to chew. If you do manage to eat them in their un-milled state, because of the dense, fibrous cell walls, you would not extract much nutrition from them. Some animals, like cows, are able to break down these "raw" grains because they have several stomachs that work on the grains over a long period of time.

Almost all grains need to be processed, in some manner, for us to eat.

<u>What are whole grains and what are refined grains?</u> There are three parts to a whole grain:
- Bran: The hard, outer layer of the grain. It contains fiber, minerals and antioxidants.
- Germ: The nutrient-rich core that contains carbs, fats, proteins, vitamins, minerals, antioxidants, and various phytonutrients. The germ is the embryo of the plant; the part that gives rise to a new plant.
- Endosperm: The biggest part of the grain, contains mostly carbs (in the form of starch) and protein.

A refined grain has had the bran and germ removed, leaving just the endosperm. Some grains, like oats, are usually eaten whole, whereas others are generally eaten refined. Many grains are consumed after they have been pulverized into very fine flour and processed into a different form. This includes wheat.

Corn is a different story. It is sold, and consumed, in a variety of forms, including: raw, dried and pulverized, cooked, and as high fructose corn syrup.

Whole grains contain the entire grain kernel — the bran, germ, and endosperm. Examples of whole grains include whole-wheat flour, bulgur (cracked wheat), oatmeal, whole cornmeal, and brown rice.

<u>Benefits of Grains</u>: Grains can be a healthy food source. In our attempts to understand, and correct, <u>metabolic syndrome</u> (obesity/weight gain, Type 2 Diabetes, hyperinsulinemia, cardio-vascular disease, among others), it is very easy to vilify grains. Even the ancient Egyptians were plagued with dental problems, cardio-vascular illness, what seems to have been diabetes, and excessive weight.

But, as the rest of this book explains, it may be more a problem of overloading, and frequency, than any inherent toxic quality of these carbs. Like most things, the dose makes the poison.

Whole grains tend to be high in many nutrients, including fiber, B vitamins, magnesium, iron, phosphorus, manganese and selenium. Some grains (like oats and whole wheat) are loaded with nutrients, whereas others (like rice and corn) are not very nutritious, even in their whole form.

- "Bran and fiber slow the breakdown of starch into glucose—thus maintaining a steady <u>blood sugar</u> rather than causing sharp spikes.

- <u>Fiber</u> helps lower cholesterol as well as move waste through the digestive tract.

- Fiber may also help prevent the formation of small blood clots that can trigger heart attacks or strokes.

- Phytochemicals and essential minerals such as magnesium, selenium and copper found in whole grains may protect against some cancers." (Harvard – School of Public Health)

Refined grains are often enriched with nutrients like iron, folate and B vitamins, to replace some of the nutrients that were lost during processing, but the phytonutrients, destroyed during processing, cannot be replaced.

Refined grains are problematical not just because they've been stripped of valuable nutrients, even if some are added back in, but also because they digest very quickly; sending a large amount of glucose into the system raising blood sugar and insulin. This may not be a problem for someone that is not insulin resistant and has a need for larger amounts of glucose (such as athletes or people doing strenuous work). The rest of us might want to proceed with caution.

Whole grains, and things like beans and chickpeas, while still high in carbs, will digest slower. This results in smaller spikes in blood sugar and insulin.

<u>Truth in Labeling</u>: I've learned to be skeptical of the food labels on processed food, especially when it comes to foods made with grain. For example, whole wheat bread sounds healthier than white bread, but is it?

According to the USDA:
- One slice of whole-wheat bread has:
    - 91 calories
    - 4 grams of protein
    - 1 gram of fat
    - 15 grams of carbohydrates
    - 2 grams of fiber

- One slice of white bread has:
    - 75 calories
    - 2 grams of protein
    - less than 1 gram of fat
    - 14 grams of carbs
    - less than 1 gram of fiber

As you can see, the differences are negligible, and you are still getting more carbs than you probably expected. You have to ask yourself if you are getting enough nutritive value to make those carbs worthwhile?

Also, while there appear to be many studies touting the benefits of whole grains, for many medical conditions, almost all of the studies are poorly done, epidemiological studies and/or paid for by food companies.

DAIRY

Dairy foods (milk and cheese) are a fairly hot topic that can get complicated quite quickly. For that reason, it has its own appendix (Appendix Dairy).

FOOD STORAGE

As you can imagine, having spent almost 20 years in the restaurant business, I'm a bit of a stickler for proper food handling, processing, and storage. While I don't date-label everything I buy, I do properly rotate food as I bring it into the house. So, since I like half-n-half in my coffee, and I hate to run out of it, I usually have one open container and two back-ups. Those get rotated from back of the fridge to the front as I use them. Anything I freeze gets labeled and dated. Now that I think of it, I do rotate everything. If I buy canned tomatoes, the new cans go toward the back of the shelf, and the old ones toward the front. I guess I automatically do that with all food stuff.

But, at this moment, I'm more concerned with the process used to store food. I'm a firm believer in stocking up when things are on sale. I have no problems with freezing meats that I'll be eating. Or buying sunflower seeds in big batches and portioning them.

One thing that has been a godsend, a truly great product that vastly extends shelf, and freezer, life, while preserving flavors and texture, has been the food vacuum sealer.

Freezer burn is gone! My sunflower seeds don't go rancid. My olive oil doesn't even get a chance to deteriorate. And my spring mix salad greens don't get funky two days after bringing them home from the store! I hate, with a passion, throwing out food and I really hate buying salad greens that start getting brown, rotting bits on them almost as soon as I get them home.

And that's where the food vacuum sealer system really pays for itself. I have a 16-cup container that will hold 16 ounces of mixed greens. There is a valve on top the lid that I attach an accessory hose to, and it sucks out all the air. I once ran an experiment by putting half of a new container of salad greens into the vacuum container and the other half I kept in its original packaging. Then I let them both sit in the fridge. After four days the greens in the original container were getting brown, nasty bits and starting to wilt. Bad enough that I would never eat it. The greens in the 16-cup container were still amazingly fresh after 21 days and, at 29 days, were just starting to wilt, but had no rotting bits.

I have smaller containers for meats (great for marinating and also keeps the fat in salami from turning rancid/oxidizing) and I store my olive oil in heavy, dark wine bottles and use vacuum seal stoppers to suck out the air. Yes, I know olive oil should be good for up to two months after opening, but as soon as it is exposed to air, it is degrading. This solves that problem!

If you to buy things in bulk, these machines are worth looking into. I recommend that you buy one with an accessory hose and get some of the associated bottle stoppers, canisters, and a few different sized bags. There are "one use" bags, but there are also zip-lock style bags that you can reseal as you use up the product. And you don't have to buy the name brand bags (which are hideously expensive). There are off-brand bags that work just as well for a fraction of the price.

PART 3: APPENDICES

Appendix RESEARCH

I know—research sounds boring. When you are the one doing it it's really kind of exciting. But reading about it can be confusing and intimidating. This appendix is my attempt to give you a basic understanding of the types of research that are done to determine whether a certain food or diet is healthy or dangerous.

Why do we do research in the first place? We do it because people tend to believe what they've heard from others, and then ignore information that contradicts that belief. We all do this—some more than others. When the scientific method was developed, about 400 years ago by Francis Bacon, it was hoped that it would help people get past their preconceived notions of what was true and provide a way to test if a certain belief really held up to reality.

While there are many types of research, we are going to focus on two:

- Observational Research
- Randomized Controlled Trials

A lot of nutritional research is classified as **"observational,"** which means it looks at the rate of a certain disease in a group of people and tries to link that disease to various lifestyle variables. In the world of nutrition, they refer to this type of research as "epidemiological" research (it has the same root as the word "epidemic," so you can think of it as the study of epidemics). Basically, the scientist observes the rate of disease in a group and also observes what other things about that group might be linked to the disease. It's really a simple form of research that sounds intimidating because it's called "epidemiological!"

Observational research is often conducted with thousands of people. One famous observational study was the Nurses' Health Study[5]. This was a study designed to look at the potential causes of chronic disease. A questionnaire was used to obtain lifestyle information, including diet, from over 100,000 women between the ages of 30 and 55. These women filled out the questionnaire every two years for about 8 years. Then, researchers looked at how many of the women developed a chronic disease (coronary heart disease, cancer, high blood pressure, etc.) and how many died of such diseases.

Then, the work of the researcher is to look back through all the questionnaire data to try to find lifestyle "links" to the various diseases.

But keep in mind the reason these studies need thousands of participants is that over a short period of time—like 8 years—not a lot of people become sick or die of these types of diseases. For example, the study reports that "of 32,317 postmenopausal women who were initially free of coronary disease, 90 women had either nonfatal myocardial infarctions (65 cases) or fatal coronary heart disease (25 cases)." So, any links identified related to heart attacks (fatal or otherwise) are based on 90 people.

It's important to point out that when an observational study finds a "link" between a lifestyle factor and a disease, that link IS NOT NECESSARILY an indication that the lifestyle factor CAUSES the disease. It might be a cause, but the limitations on how observational data are collected and how they can be analyzed prevent the researcher (and the rest of us) from knowing if it is an actual cause. So, when a research study says it found a LINK between a lifestyle factor and a disease, it's really saying it found a POSSIBLE cause of the disease.

The reason we can't know for sure if a particular lifestyle factor (let's call it Factor X) causes the disease is because there could be other factors that influence Factor X. These "other factors" could be things that were measured in the study itself, or things that the researchers didn't think of—or have the budget—to include.

If you can't prove cause, why use this type of research? Well, compared to the type of research that CAN provide insights as to the cause of an illness, observational research is much cheaper. It's also a way to identify specific factors to study in the more expensive research. Observational studies allow you to look for links (potential causes) across hundreds of lifestyle variables at the same time. You can then spend the big bucks testing the potential causes that seem most promising. But, as you will see later, the big-buck studies can only test one link at a time. So, testing hundreds of lifestyle factors one at a time is just too costly.

A more powerful type of research is a **Randomized Controlled Trial** (RCT). The strength of a Randomized Controlled Trial comes from a couple of aspects of this type of research.

First, an RCT focuses on a **single factor** thought to possibly cause the disease of interest. As a running example, let's say that from observational research, we saw that smoking cigarettes was linked to lung cancer. That is, let's say that in an observational study we saw that people who had lung cancer were more likely to be smokers than were people without lung cancer. So now we want to see if we can determine if smoking causes lung cancer.

To do this, we need to set up an experiment. We need to get two groups of people, Group Test and Group Control. We'll start with 100 non-smokers and form the two groups from these 100 non-smokers. Group Test (50 people) will be told to smoke cigarettes and Group Control (50 people) will be told not to smoke. Of course, we could never conduct such an experiment due to ethical concerns, but it makes for a clear example. (This is why so much research on deadly diseases are done on animals like mice and rats—you can assign lab animals to dangerous conditions.)

We form the groups by assigning people to one of the two groups randomly. Randomly assigning people to one of the two groups works to balance each group on factors such as age, gender, income, employment status, education level, eating habits and other factors we might not know about.

Next, we monitor the people in each group to make sure people in the Test Group are smoking and the people in the Control Group are not smoking.

After a period of time, we look to see how many people in each group have developed lung cancer. If a significantly greater number in the Test Group have lung cancer, we can conclude that lung cancer is caused by smoking. We can assume this because we randomly assigned people to the groups and controlled for other factors except for smoking. Since the only thing different between the two groups was whether the members smoked or not, smoking must have been a cause of the lung cancer.

Now, if there were people in the Control Group that also had lung cancer, we would need to conclude that smoking was **one** cause of lung cancer, but that there are likely other causes.

RCTs are typically conducted with small groups of people because of the expense to conduct the study. But because of the tight controls of other factors, extremely large samples aren't needed.

Unfortunately, when the media report on research studies, they often don't appreciate the difference between an Observational study and a Randomized Controlled Trial. A recent observational study that found a **link** between red meat and cancer was reported in the media as "New study says red meat causes cancer!" But the study just reported a link—they did not determine that a causal relationship exists between red meat and cancer. This is, obviously, an important distinction! So, when you see media reports of Factor X causes Disease Y, read the study details. Most news articles will post a link to the original study, so you can look how the study was done. Did they randomly assign people to groups? If not, it wasn't the powerful type of study that can determine a cause and effect relationship.

The reason eggs were bad for you at one point in time and fine for you later was that the "eggs are bad for you" was based on observational research. Once tested in RCTs, they were found to be safe. (In fact, eggs were deemed bad because of their cholesterol content—and cholesterol had been thought to be linked to heart disease. But it turns out that cholesterol is not bad for you.)

Another aspect of research to be aware of is the term "statistical significance." You might see a study that says something like "People taking Treatment X were less likely to die of a heart attack than those taking Treatment Y, at a statistically significant level." Here's what that is referring to:

Experiments following the scientific method start with what's called a "null hypothesis"—it is often referred to as the hypothesis of no difference and is denoted as "H_0." When a scientist wants to test, say, the difference between the effectiveness of a low-fat diet versus a low-carb diet in terms of weight loss, H_0 (the null hypothesis) is that there will be no difference between the 2 diets—if people are randomly assigned to one of the diets, the average weight loss in the Low-fat Group will be the same as the average weight loss in the Low-carb Group. The scientist would then conduct the experiment (maybe have each group eat their assigned diet for 12 months). Then the scientist would weigh everyone and compare their weights to what they weighed just before starting their assigned diet.

The way statistical tests appropriate for this type of experiment work, is that they test if the H_0 is true. In our example, the test would compare the average weight loss of the two groups in light of how much the weight of people in each Group varied. If the statistical test shows that the difference between the two Groups is "statistically significant," it means we can reject H_0 and conclude that the two diets performed differently with respect to weight loss. If the statistical test shows that the difference between the two Groups is NOT "statistically significant," it means we **cannot** reject H_0 and must conclude that the two diets performed equally with respect to weight loss.

But no experiment is perfect, so we allow scientists to be 95% sure when it comes to rejecting H_0. That's why you would see—if you delved into the research done in the area—many studies testing the same thing. Sometimes the tests change the type of people being tested, or the percentage of carbs (for our example) in the diet, etc. Seeing many studies concluding the same thing (each with 95% surety) gives us more confidence that conclusion is right. That's how science works. If you saw the results of 20 tests of Drug X versus a placebo (a pill the same shape as the drug but with no active ingredients in it) and 10 times the people taking the drug did better and 10 times people taking the placebo did better, you might not have a lot of confidence that Drug X was effective. You'd likely be more confident in Drug X if 18 of the 20 tests showed people taking Drug X did better.

Appendix INSULIN

The body has two separate systems for communicating with its different parts:
- The Nervous System: the network of cells and fibers that transmits electric impulses between parts of the body.
- The Endocrine System: A chemical messenger system that maintains feedback loops of hormones released directly into the bloodstream, that regulates body functions, tissues, organs and cells.

Insulin is part of the endocrine system and is produced in the pancreas. Insulin does three important things within the body related to metabolism. First, it transports glucose to cells within the body and interacts with receptors on cell membranes that allow glucose into the cells. The cells then use glucose molecules to produce the energy they need to work (and for us to live). Insulin also plays a similar role with muscle and liver cells and glycogen (a dense form of glucose)—allowing muscle and liver cells to store glycogen for later use. The third role is a similar role, this time with liver cells and fat cells (adipose tissue)—allowing these cells to store fat.

Insulin is secreted by the pancreas into the bloodstream when we eat carbohydrates and proteins. Insulin is what our body uses to regulate the amount of glucose in our blood. Too much glucose in our blood is dangerous—so if you eat a lot of carbohydrates in a meal, your pancreas secretes a lot of insulin to help transport the glucose to cells. When the cells that use glucose are full, insulin will take glycogen to the liver and muscle cells for storage. When the glycogen storage locations are full, insulin takes fatty acids to the liver and fat cells for storage. While you eat and for 2 to 4 hours (on average) after you eat, the heightened level of insulin in the blood (the level achieved as a reaction to eating) stops the body from using fat for energy and stores some of what we eat as body fat.

There is always a "base level" of insulin in the blood (if your pancreas is working; Type 1 diabetes is what they call the condition when a person's pancreas doesn't produce insulin). If this base level isn't too high, the glucagon in the bloodstream (also produced by the pancreas) will get your body to start burning fat for energy.

Appendix THE CASE AGAINST PROCESSED CARBS

In addition to the impact carbohydrates in general have on the production of insulin, eating processed carbs causes even more insulin secretion.

The carbs that get "processed" are typically grains. Grains are forms of grass. We use the kernels (the seeds of the plant) to make things like bread. Before processing, a whole grain kernel (we'll use wheat as an example) has three parts: The bran, the germ and the endosperm. (Also, see "Healthy" Whole Grains in Part 2 of the book where Evan goes into more detail on grains.)

In a sense, a kernel of grain is like an egg: The bran is the outer skin of the edible kernel—like the shell of an egg, but you can eat the covering of a grain. It contains antioxidants, B vitamins and fiber. The germ is the part of the seed that has the potential to grow into a new plant—like the yolk of an egg. It also contains many B vitamins, some protein, minerals, and healthy fats. The endosperm is the germ's food supply—like the egg white. The endosperm provides energy to the growing plant so it can create roots as well as push itself through the ground to get sunlight. The endosperm is the biggest part of the kernel. It contains starchy carbohydrates, proteins and small amounts of vitamins and minerals.

When a kernel of wheat is processed, the bran and germ are removed and discarded, so all that's left is the endosperm. This is done because the bran can be hard for some people to digest and the oils in the germ can cause the flour made from the grain to spoil. Flour made from only the endosperm can last for months or years (when ultra-processed) without spoiling. The white flour is also fluffy when cooked so food companies can use less in their products.

You will often see white flour or white bread tout they are enriched with vitamins and minerals. That's because the vitamins and minerals are stripped away from the kernel when the bran and germ are discarded—so the manufacturer needs to add them back in at the end of the process if the product is going to have any nutrient value besides providing non-essential glucose to the body.

The difference in our insulin response to eating processed grains versus whole grain products is dramatic. Research[32] shows we can secrete twice as much insulin in response to processed wheat versus whole-grain wheat. This is why I stay away from processed grains as much as possible.

Appendix LCHF (Low-Carb/High-Fat)

There are a lot of studies showing the benefits of a low-carb diet on heart-health risk factors. A review of 23 separate reports was published in 2012[23] that showed the low-carb diet to be associated with significant weight loss, lower body mass index, smaller abdominal circumference, lower blood pressure, lower triglyceride levels in the blood, lower fasting blood sugar and insulin levels and an increase in high-density lipoprotein (HDL or "good") cholesterol.

You've seen *how* and *why* the LCHF diet works. Here, several questions and concerns are presented:

Q: Do you need to stay on the LCHF diet the rest of your life to get the effects.
A: Of course, the answer is yes. It's "of course yes" because we are dealing with how the human body has evolved to react to carbohydrates—and, more importantly, how your body reacts to carbs. Human's reactions to carbohydrates might evolve

further to the point where a high intake of carbs isn't a problem. But your reaction carbohydrates won't change—all you can do is adapt to the environment given the genes you have by lowering your intake of carbs.

This type of life-time adaptation isn't unusual in our lives. For example, if you stop taking a medication for allergy symptoms, the symptoms come back. But you don't think of the medication as not working. It's the same with a LCHF diet. It will help you get and stay lean—but you have to eat a LCHF diet for it to work!

How low you have to go with carbs might change. I started going very low but have seen, with time, that I can handle more than the 20 grams of carbs (30 or 35) without gaining weight.

Q: How low do I need to take my carbs?
A: There is no one answer to this question. It really depends on your body and your goals. I seem to be very sensitive to carbs. When I started on a strict low-carb approach, I was 278 pounds*. I wanted to lose 80 pounds. So, I cut back to 20 grams of net carbs. The magic number—where most people start to see weight loss—is keeping net carbs under 100 grans/day. Your results may vary.

Q: How quickly will I start to lose weight?
A: That depends on several factors, such as how overweight you are now and how low you take your carbs. Gender plays a role too, because estrogen plays a role in weight control. The key is to remember that you are NOT a machine. Be patient as your body learns to live with fewer carbs.

I'm a geek and love data, so I weight myself every day. If you want to do this, be sure to weigh yourself at a consistent point in the day (I weigh myself after my "morning routine"). Of course, if you wear clothes when you weigh yourself, what you wear will impact the measurement on the scale. If you do this, you will see that there will be times where it seems that what you've eaten the day before has no correlation to how much you weigh the next day! There have been days I've kept my net carbs to 20 grams, and I've lost a quarter of a pound; other days, I've gained a half a pound. Stress, the amount of sleep you get, even the weather can impact how your

[* I had lost about 100 pounds by inadvertently lowering my carbs on a point-system diet—I saw I could eat more protein if I ate less carbs. But I didn't measure or track what I ate, so I don't know how low my carbs were then. I can confidently say they weren't as low as 20 net grams per day!]

body reacts to the food you eat. Be patient. Look at and feel how your clothes fit you. Soon the jean you had to suck in to close will fit without a second thought.

Q: Will I get all my vitamins and minerals from a LCHF diet?
A: You will if you eat a range of foods—just like you would need to on the USDA-recommended dietary guidelines. Leafy greens are a good source for Vitamin A, C, E and K. Meat and fish are good sources of B-complex and D. All these foods are mineral-rich, as well. Some people on a LCHF diet take vitamin supplements, but I haven't taken them yet.

Q: Is a LCHF diet safe? Even for kids?
A: There have been no known deaths linked to the LCHF diet. Remember, there are NO ESSENTIAL DIETARY CARBOHYDRATES. If you (or a child) never ate another carbohydrate again, and you ate a healthy mix of other foods (you might need vitamin/mineral supplements if you weren't eating a single gram of carbs), there is no reason to believe you would live a day less. The body will make all the glucose it needs from dietary or body fat.

Q: How does the LCHF diet compare to a low-fat diet in terms of weight loss?
A: A recent review of 62 Randomized Controlled Trials[9] (the strongest form or research, which allows you to determine causation) by the UK's Public Health Collaboration found the following: Of the studies showing a significant difference, 31 favored the low-carb diet (people on low-carb lost more weight); 0 favored the low-fat diet. The other tests didn't show a statistical difference between the two—but of these other 31 tests (that didn't show a statistically significant difference) 22 favored the low-carb diet, 7 favored the low-fat diet, and for 2 studies, the amount of weight loss was exactly the same.

All in all, the low-carb diet has been shown to result in more weight loss than the low-fat diet.

Appendix ONE MAN'S EGO

We have evidence as far back as 1863[33] that obesity was treated with a low-carb/high-fat diet. Why, then, did we end up with a low-fat/high carb diet recommendation from the USDA?

After World War 1, the rate of heart disease started to increase. Researchers started looking for what was causing this rise. One man, Ancel Keys, suspected the culprit was dietary fat. On the face of it, it sounds like a logical cause—you get a heart attack and your coronary arteries are clogged with a fatty substance, like the clogged drain of a kitchen sink. It seemed to make sense that it was coming from the fat you eat. But it's not wise to just say something is true because it makes sense. You need to do research and show that your theory is correct.

Keys had a bachelor's degree in economics and a PhD in marine biology. He worked as a professor at the University of Minnesota studying fish physiology. He also had an interest in human physiology and conducted some nutrition-oriented research around the end of World War 2. In fact, if you've ever heard of the military food kits soldiers were given back then referred to as K-Rations, the "K" is for Keys, who developed them.

In the early 1950s, Keys published a paper in the newsletter of Mt. Sinai Hospital, in New York City, that he said proved his theory that dietary fat caused heart disease. He presented data from various countries showing a strong relationship between fat in the diet and deaths from heart disease.

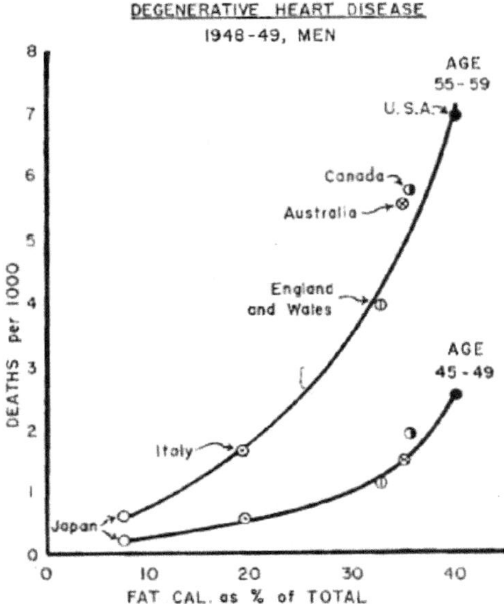

FIG. 2. Mortality from degenerative heart disease (categories 93 and 94 in the Revision of 1938, categories 420 and 422 in the Revision of 1948, International List. National vital statistics from official sources. Fat calories as percentage of total calories calculated from national food balance data for 1949 supplied by the Nutrition Division, Food and Agriculture Organization of the United Nations.

The graph above does, indeed, show a strong relationship between dietary fat and death from heart disease! What some other researchers pointed out, however, was that Keys didn't show <u>all</u> the data he had at his disposal. When you show the data from all the countries that were studied, the story is a little different:

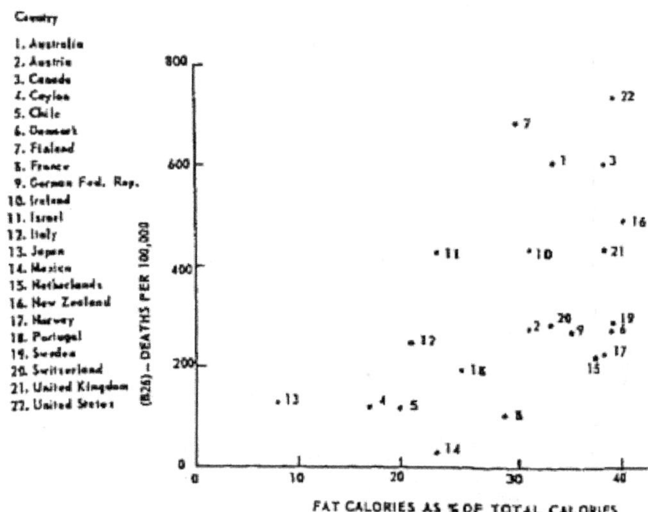

Fig. 3. Mortality from arteriosclerotic and degenerative heart disease (B-26) and fat calories as per cent of total calories in males fifty-five to fifty-nine years. Calculated from national food balance data by F.A.O. (see text for definition).

Keys essentially "cherry-picked" only the data that fit his theory. This is the exact opposite of how science is supposed to work. As a scientist, if you test your theory and if the data don't support it, you change your theory. For Keys, the data didn't support his theory, so he changed the data.

As a means of deflecting the exposure of his fraud, he then said it was **saturated** fat in the diet that caused heart disease. In the meantime, he managed to get on the nutrition committee at the American Heart Association, where he pushed hard to get a low-fat diet recommended for the American public. And he got his way—it was largely his influence that resulted in the food pyramid being based in grains/carbohydrates with fats and oils at the top to be used sparingly.

Fortunately, research on fats didn't stop then. Dozens of studies have been done in this area. If you are interested in even more details on this body of research, I highly recommend a book by Nina Teicholz called The Big Fat Surprise (see recommended reading list).

One analysis of data for various countries actually shows the rate of death from heart disease goes down with the amount of saturated fat consumed. Not to spoil Nina's surprise, but it turns out (based on dozens and dozens of studies) that eating fat doesn't make you fat!

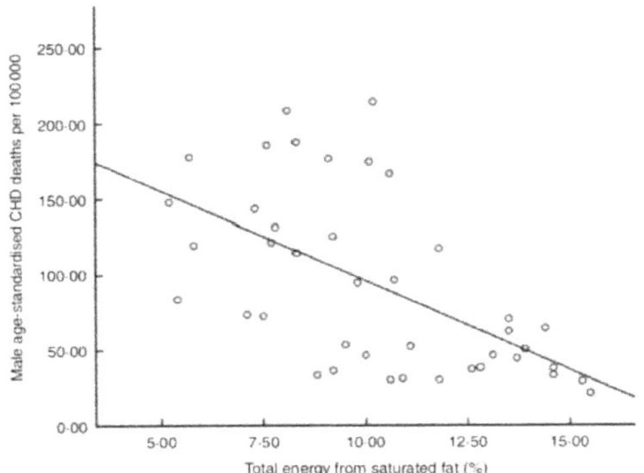

Remember how it is insulin that regulates the generation and storage of body fat—and how it blocks the use of body fat for energy when levels are high? Insulin levels rise when you eat carbohydrates—not when you eat fat. Excess sugar in your blood will get converted to fat and stored in your fat cells—that blood sugar comes from carbs. Yes—if you eat fatty foods along with a high level of carbs, the fat you eat will end up as body fat. But the fat you eat on a low-carb diet gets used for energy and does not get stored as fat, because on a low-carb diet, insulin levels can stay low (since there isn't so much sugar in your blood).

Despite the facts, however, Keys got his way and America was put on a low-fat diet. The thing is, people tend to self-regulate how much protein they eat (relative to what their energy needs are). So, if you ate 2000 calories a day before going low-fat and you stay at 2000 calories on a low-fat diet, chances are, you will raise your carbs—to the levels suggested by the food pyramid. It's that high level of carbs that can trigger the hormonal imbalance that leads to obesity.

Why hasn't anyone said "Hey, we goofed on that one! Go back to eating fat!" Well, personally, I think there are companies in the food industry making too much money off of low-fat food and companies in the pharmaceutical industry making too much money off of high-fat people. I mean, consider: Type 2 diabetes is the body's inability to regulate blood sugar; blood sugar comes largely from carbohydrates in the diet. But the treatment for Type 2 diabetes is to have people inject more insulin to deal with all the carbs they are eating instead of just eating fewer carbs (which would lead to less sugar in the blood that needs regulating).

Appendix FAT

As you read in Appendix ONE MAN'S EGO, fat got a bad name based on an idea—eating fat clogged one's arteries and caused heart attacks. This idea is called The Lipid (fat) Hypothesis or The Diet/Heart Hypothesis. The idea was that A) if you ate too much fat (saturated fat, specifically) your cholesterol would go up; B) the high cholesterol would lead to plaque building up in your arteries (think grease in the pipes of your kitchen sink) and eventually block the blood flow to the point you had a heart attack.

Admittedly, the idea seems reasonable. It just happens to **NOT** be true. It would be somewhat comforting to know that everyone just assumed this idea was true and developed plans accordingly to ensure our health. Unfortunately, this happens to **NOT** be true, as well. After Ancel Keys (the man with the ego) published his seven-country study in support of the Lipid Hypothesis, researchers exposed his fraudulent report for what it was. But people in high places listened to Keys and not the evidence.

For decades, fat was seen as bad—and is still seen that way by many people including those in the fields of medicine and nutrition. This led to the USDA dietary recommendations of a low-fat diet. Given people can only tolerate a certain level of protein at any given meal, if you reduce the fat, you end up adding carbohydrates. The low-fat dietary recommendation spawned a huge sector in the food industry—Low-Fat Foods. But just like with a meal, if you make a food product low-fat, you need to add carbohydrates. And as we've seen, high levels of carbohydrates can lead to heart attacks: the low-fat, "heart-healthy" food on the market are not really heart-healthy.

The question remains, however, is fat any healthier? The answer is yes. To explain why the answer is Fat is healthy, let's look at the two main points of the Lipid Hypothesis and what the research evidence is for each part.

A) Does eating fat raise your cholesterol? No. A well-controlled study[24] looking at the effects of a low-carb/high fat diet on cholesterol noted that HDL (good) cholesterol went up and LDL (bad) cholesterol went down. So, eating fat a high-fat diet actually improves your cholesterol numbers.

B) Does high cholesterol lead to heart attacks?   No. A research study conducted in 1966[25] concluded that there was no evidence that high cholesterol shortens the life span. Another study from 1991[26], among people aged 60 – 74 showed that having very high cholesterol was associated with a *lower* risk of death from a heart attack or any other cause. This was confirmed 10 years later[27] in an analysis of data from the Honolulu Heart Study.

Then why all the fuss about cholesterol? That's a good question! One place to look are the studies related to a class of drugs called statins. Statins are drugs that lower your cholesterol. Pharmaceutical companies worked with researchers (that is, the pharmaceutical companies paid for the research) to study the impact of statins on cholesterol and the rate of heart disease. The basic study design is that you start with people with high cholesterol and randomly assign them to one of two groups: The Test Group gets the statin; the Control Group gets a placebo (a sugar pill). Then they look at the cholesterol level of each group and the rate of death from heart disease (heart attacks).

If you look at one of the original ads for Lipitor, they said their research showed a 36% reduction in heart events (either a fatal or non-fatal heart attack) when comparing the two groups. But in the fine print, they tell the truth—they show that 2% of those in the Test Group had a fatal or non-fatal heart attack (it was actually 1.9%[4] but they rounded up) while 3% of the Control Group had a similar attack. To most of us, that would be a 1.1% reduction in the rate of heart attack. But that doesn't sound as good as 36%. So, the drug company took the 1.1% difference between the two groups and divided it by the 3% of the Control Group and got 36%. That, ladies and gentlemen, is how you deceive with statistics.

Now, maybe a lower rate of a heart attack in 1 out of 100 people are odds you like. Just keep in mind that there are a lot of side-effects from use of statins, including an increased risk of Type 2 diabetes—which can result in heart disease!

In summary, research shows that fat is not bad for us like people have led us to believe. In fact, the evidence points to the benefits of a low-carb/high-fat diet.

Appendix FRUIT

We've all been told that fruit is healthy for us and that we should eat a lot of it. We are told fruit is rich in vitamins and minerals. And while fruit does contain vitamins and minerals, so do protein and fats. In fact, you can get all the vitamins a body needs from meat, fish and eggs (you need to eat the organ meats of animals to get vitamin C, but it's there!).

We evolved, over millions of years, with access to fruit and vegetables on a seasonal basis. We ate fruit when it was ripe on the tree. Our ancient ancestors didn't have apples flown in from New Zealand and other parts of the world all year round. And we didn't cultivate fruit trees until relatively recently (in our history). It's the same with vegetables—we just ate what we found. Fruits and vegetables weren't a big part of our diet (in terms of percentage of calories eaten) for the first 99.9% of our history.

The bad thing about fruit is that it is high in fructose (a natural sugar). Fructose is interesting in that it does not create a high insulin response. Instead, it gets sent straight to the liver and stored as fat. That's why High Fructose Corn Syrup ends up being so fattening.

Appendix TALKING TO DOCTORS

Talking to doctors about a low-carb/high-fat diet can be challenging. Some doctors are fully on board with such a diet and understand how it works with, instead of against, our physiology. Some are even treating their Type 2 diabetic patients with a low-carb/high-fat diet.

Others are more resistant. I've had people tell me that their doctor said an LCHF diet would kill them by putting them into ketosis. That doctor was likely confusing ketosis with diabetic ketoacidosis. Most people go into some level of ketosis every night when they sleep. You need a non-working pancreas to go into diabetic ketoacidosis.

I don't think doctors are trying to keep you from getting lean—I think they are genuinely concerned for your health. It's just that some haven't stopped to look at the more recent RCT research (see Appendix RESEARCH) on the topic or they just don't have a firm understanding of human physiology as it relates to weight management (a lot of the current understanding in this area is also very recent).

If you get resistance from your doctor when you discuss a LCHF approach to eating, one thing you could do is make a deal: try the LCHF approach for say, 6 months and compare your blood test results. One thing you will find in the blood test results after 6 months of eating LCHF is your LDL cholesterol will likely have gone up. But don't worry. When you do your cholesterol test, ask for the LDL particle size counts. What you will likely find is that you will have more of the "Pattern A" LDL (large, fluffy particles) which are not a problem—it's the small, dense LDL particles (Pattern B) that are the problem[21].

Side Note: **Ketoacidosis** *is a condition in which the process of making ketones is unregulated—this can happen to Type 1 diabetics because their pancreas never produces insulin, and it is insulin that keeps the production of ketones in check (insulin does a lot of jobs).*

Ketone levels in the blood can be measured with a monitor like those used by diabetics to measure their blood sugar. Someone who eats a lot of carbs will have ketone levels at or almost at zero. On my low-carb/high-fat diet, where I try to eat no more than 20 grams of carbs a day (4% of my calories), my blood ketone levels average around 0.6 mmol/L (millimoles per liter)—a level considered to be "nutritional ketosis."

If someone is on a medically controlled "ketogenic diet" because of treatment for epilepsy, under hospital control, they might reach a level of 3 or even 5 mmol/L—but this would take incredible levels of care as to the proteins and fats the patient was given in addition to limiting or eliminating carbs from the diet.

When someone's pancreas fails to work and ketone production becomes unregulated, that persons level of ketones in the blood reaches 30 mmol/L or more— that's ketoacidosis. That's why Type 1 diabetics need to take insulin—their pancreas doesn't produce insulin, so they need to inject it. Eating a low-carb diet will not put you into ketoacidosis.

Appendix ADULTS ONLY

This Appendix deals with a practice that **children 18 and under should not do—** it's the practice of fasting. Fasting is something humans have done since the first of us walked on the planet. It is misunderstood by many, so I'll start with a bit of background.

Fasting is NOT starvation. **Starvation** is the uncontrolled withholding of food. The key word being "uncontrolled." People are starved as punishment or due to food shortages beyond their control—they don't know when or where their next meal is coming from.

Fasting is the controlled withholding of food. You can think of fasting as just "not eating." You aren't eating but you know where to get food and you control when you eat next.

We all fast every day when we sleep. During that time, our bodies have a chance to metabolize body fat for energy. How much fat a person burns depends on their weight, the timing of their last meal and their resting (or "fasted") insulin level. If a person's insulin response is normal—that is, if they are not insulin resistant—and they didn't have a snack before going to bed, they will burn fat nearly the entire time they are asleep. Granted, it's not a lot of calories, but a 150-pound person could lose up to 2 ounces of body fat per night if they get 8 hours of sleep. Not bad for just sleeping. And that adds up to almost a pound a week.

Unfortunately for people (like me) who are insulin resistant, that weight—and more—is gained back the next day.

The idea of fasting as a weight-loss technique is to extend the not-eating period to allow the body more time to metabolize (use as fuel) stored fat. Remember, once we start metabolizing fat, we don't stop using it as fuel until we eat—which triggers the pancreas to start putting insulin in your blood, which in turn stops the fat-metabolizing hormone (glucagon) from doing its job. The insulin, then, puts the priority on burning glucose from the carbs we just ate.

The overall idea of fasting is so simple it sometimes confuses people! The idea is just that you don't eat. That said, while fasting, experts recommend that you drink water when you are thirsty. Drinking coffee or tea (without cream or sugar) can also be taken without breaking your fast. Be careful if you use a capsule coffee/tea machine, however, because some of the capsuled beverages contain sugar.

Types of fasting: There are two basic types of fasting—Intermittent Fasting (IF) and Extended Fasting (EF). The difference between the two types is just the length of the fasting period.

IF is easy to do and there are several schedules to choose from (or you can make your own). Some are named for the length of the fasting period and what's called the "eating window," or the period of time in which you eat food. You don't eat during the entire eating window, but you fit your meals within that eating window time period.

The IF schedule I like is called 16:8 fasting. I fast for 16 hours and then eat my meals within an 8-hour window. I eat 2 low-carb/high-fat meals a day—lunch (around 1:00PM) and dinner (around 8:00PM). I typically finish dinner sometime before 9:00PM—so that's what I consider the start of my fasting period. From 9:00PM one day until 1:00PM the next, I don't eat. I only take water and black coffee. So, I basically just skip the morning meal (which is when most people *break* their *fast*!). Importantly, no snacks during the fasting period.

When you start this type of fasting schedule, you'll get hungry in the morning the first 4 or 5 days. This is because your body gets used to a schedule and a hormone called ghrelin gets released to remind you it's your usual mealtime. But your body will learn that you aren't doing a morning meal anymore and it will stop making your stomach growl and feeling hungry.

My eating window is from 1:00PM to 9:00PM. I tend to eat a fuller meal for lunch and a lighter meal for dinner—but that's personal preference. I also choose NOT to snack between meals to give my pancreas more of a rest after lunch. Of course, I'm keeping my carbs low, but I'm insulin resistant so my body is more sensitive to snacking. If I do eat a snack, I go for something high in fat like macadamia nuts.

Other IF schedules include 20:4 (sometimes called One Meal A Day or OMAD), 18:6, and 5:2 (which refers to 5 days of eating and 2 days of fasting per week—you schedule the eating days and fasting days as you like). As I write this book, I'm doing something called Alternate Day Fasting (ADF). With ADF, I fast from my usual after-dinner hour of 9:00PM until lunch two days later. So, if I start the fast after dinner on Sunday, I don't eat again until lunch on Tuesday.

Anything longer than ADF is considered Extended Fasting (EF). EF just extends the fasting period. I've done two EFs of just over 80 hours. I started my first 80+-hour fast on a Sunday evening and didn't eat again until Thursday—but I ate a morning meal that day, I didn't wait until lunch.

Once your body gets used to NOT expecting food at any given point during the day or any given day during the week, you barely notice you are fasting. The big thing you do notice is how much extra time you have since you aren't cooking, eating or cleaning up afterwards.

But these extended fasts are really only for those looking to lose weight. **If you are underweight, pregnant, breastfeeding or prone to eating disorders, EF is NOT recommended**.

Both Intermittent Fasting and Extended Fasting can be used to lose weight and help stabilize your weight once you reach your goal. It's a different approach to dieting as it just cuts out food altogether. And it turns out that's why it is so effective.

Side Note: One of the big myths regarding fasting is that if you fast you will lose a lot lean muscle mass. This, however, is not true. If you think about it, humans would not have survived periods of food shortages if, when we didn't eat, our bodies turned to our muscles for energy. This would be, for lack of a better word, stupid—given the fat we all have stored on our bodies that, gram per gram, provide over two times the energy as the protein our muscles could provide, and the fact that we would have needed our muscles to get more food.

Why the Advice the Doctor Gives You to Lose Weight Typically Doesn't Work (for context, I have repeated these first few pages from earlier in the book)

If you've ever been overweight, your doctor probably advised you to lose weight by eating less and getting some exercise. The "eat less/move more" approach has been prescribed for weight loss for decades. Typically, it works well at first. You cut back on the food you eat and go to the gym or walk more—and you start to lose weight. Then after a few months your weight loss slows down, and then it stalls. Soon after, even though you are watching what you eat and exercising, you start gaining weight!

Then, if you are like me, you give up, only to start the same process after a year or so. And, of course, everyone blames you for not having the willpower to stick to the plan.

This cycle happens to almost everyone who tries it. Why? The "eat less/move more" approach to weight loss is based on the belief that the amount of energy going into your body (the amount of food you eat) and the amount of energy your body uses, are independent of each other—that is, it is assumed that you can lower the amount of energy going into the body without impacting the amount of energy your body uses.

This belief is just wrong[18].

Our bodies regulate our weight like they regulate our temperature. If we get too hot, we sweat to cool ourselves down; when we are too cold, we shiver to warm up. And we do these things automatically—they are really beyond our conscious control. For example, if we are out on a hot, humid day, we can't keep ourselves from sweating.

A similar thing happens with your weight—especially when you primarily metabolize (burn) carbs for energy. First, I'll describe how the weight regulation system works. Then I'll explain what happens when the system is running primarily on glucose (the sugar from carbs).

The full explanation of the regulatory system for weight is much too complex for this book. If you are interested in the full story, check out "The Physiology of Body Weight Regulation"[12]. Our understanding of the full story is still being researched— more is learned each year as more research is done. The article I just referenced strays a bit from what I've presented here, but their discussion of some of the hormonal and enzyme regulators of weight are on target. And while it is, to a large extent, an overview, the article contains further references if you want to go even deeper.

The simplified weight-regulation system looks like this:

Your body needs a certain amount of energy to run on each day to live. We talk about this amount of energy in terms of calories (it's actually kilocalories, but we just call it calories). You can look online for "Basal Metabolic Rate" charts that show how many calories, on average, a man or a woman needs, per day, to function given their height and weight. For me, it's 2165. That means that if my insulin levels and response to food are normal, and I eat 2165 calories a day, my weight will stay stable. How does that work since I don't know, day-to-day, how many calories I'm eating **or** using?!

Your body keeps track of your energy. Not in terms of calories—there is no calorie counter in your brain. But if you are "insulin-normal" (that is, if your insulin levels and response are normal, and all the other hormones that regulate weight are normal) your brain understands your current energy balance. But it's not something you are directly conscious of—it's one of those systems that work in the background, like temperature control[13][14].

If the weight-control system in my body is working correctly, and I eat 2300 calories instead of 2165, my body would get me to move more than usual—I might get fidgety or feel like going for a long walk[15]. Or I might just get a little warmer if I resist moving more since we burn calories to create body heat. I'm not consciously aware that my body is trying to work off those extra calories, but that's what it's doing. The system wants to maintain an energy balance.

If I move too little (if I use fewer than 2165 calories), my body will send me signals that I don't need to eat so much—I might skip a meal "because I just don't feel hungry" or I will get full sooner than usual, before finishing my meal—or I'll decide to just eat a small meal. Again, the system wants to maintain an energy balance.

Here is the reason the Eat Less/Move More diets DON'T typically work long-term[16]:

Let's say that for my attempt to lose weight, I cut back to 1865 calories a day—a 300 calorie per day "deficit," as they say in the diet industry. Does my body notice this? You bet it does! If I eat 1865 calories instead of 2165, I'll get hungrier and want to eat more—my body wants me to hit that 2165 calorie energy balance target. My conscious brain knows I want to lose weight, but the subconscious brain doesn't know—it's an automatic system.

Okay, but I do know I want to lose weight, so I can decide to live with the hunger. If I do that, my body responds by lowering my Basal Metabolism—that is, it slows me down, so I don't use up as much energy. It can take a few weeks for this to happen. But it will happen. If I eat 1865 calories a day, eventually, by body will slow me down so I only use 1865 calories a day. I'll find myself driving to the store instead of walking. I'll sit in front of the TV instead of going for that bike ride. It's an automatic system that tries to balance the energy used based on the energy coming in.

And "moving more" makes the calorie deficit worse! If I'm eating 1865 calories and burning an extra 300 at the gym, I have a 600 calorie per day deficit. After a month or so, what had been good weight loss progress will start to slow down—because my body is trying to balance the energy going out to what's coming in.

Worse yet, my body will remember I used to weigh more[17]. To help me gain back the weight I lost, it lowers my basal metabolism so much that even at a 600-calorie deficit from the 2165 I used to eat, I gain weight. So, while I'm eating 1865 and exercising to an effective rate of 1565 calories per day (a 600-calorie deficit from my original 2165), my body will slow down to maybe 1365—so I start gaining weight. I can try to fight this process and exercise even more and eat even less, but in the end I'll be so hungry and tired all the time I'll end up eating more and exercising less, and I'll gain all the weight back—just like my body wants. You can see why Dr. Jason Fung, in his book "The Obesity Code," says "the caloric-reduction theory of obesity was as useful as a half-built bridge."[19]

Now, in a body that is insulin resistant (like mine and many overweight or obese people) the problem is amplified. It's amplified because we don't have access to the stored energy from fat, or from all the food we eat after we eat it, because insulin stops the usage of body fat for fuel and puts a lot of the excess potential energy from the food we eat into our fat cells (which stays there because our insulin levels are always high enough to halt the production of the fat-burning hormone, glucagon).

So, if the chart says I should eat 2165 calories a day and I measure and eat 2165 calories exactly, but my resting insulin level is high, my body will see that as a deficit—because not all 2165 calories will be available to me. Because of the high insulin levels in my blood, some of the energy from those calories will be stored and trapped in my fat cells. As I mentioned earlier in the book, this is why overweight/obese people are always hungry and/or don't move a lot. It's because to their body, they are restricting the calories available when they eat the "recommended" number of calories—so their weight-control system makes them want to eat more calories and/or use less energy.

The overweight person is responding to the same signals the lean person is. When a lean person's body recognizes a deficit in calories, it makes the lean person hungry and gets them thinking about food. The same thing happens with overweight and obese people. To the outside world it LOOKS like the overweight person is overeating when they have their second Big Mac. But the part of the obese person's subconscious energy-balance system that "sees" how much energy is available to them doesn't see all of the first Big Mac—so it sends signals to eat more. And these signals are no more under the control of the overweight person than anyone's ability to not sweat on a hot, humid day.

Does Fasting Work the Same Way?

No! It turns out that our bodies react differently to eating less (a calorie-deficit diet) than it does to not eating at all (fasting).

And, as you've seen, our bodies can use a body-fat (fatty acids) as well as glucose to function. While much of our body can run on fatty acids directly our brain cannot. But our brain CAN use an energy source derived from fat: ketone bodies. When we are metabolizing ketone bodies, it's called being in ketosis.

But don't worry! While many people—even many doctors—confuse ketosis with diabetic ketoacidosis, they are in fact 2 very different things.

Ketoacidosis is a condition in which the process of making ketones is unregulated—this can happen to Type 1 diabetics because their pancreas never produces insulin, and it is insulin that keeps the production of ketones in check (insulin does a lot of jobs).

Ketones levels in the blood can be measured with a monitor like those used by diabetics to measure their blood sugar. Someone who eats a lot of carbs will have ketone levels at or almost at zero. On my low-carb/high-fat diet, where I try to eat no more than 20 grams of carbs a day (4% of my calories), my blood ketone levels average around 0.6 mmol/L (millimoles per liter)—a level considered to be "nutritional ketosis."

If someone is on a medically controlled "ketogenic diet" because of treatment for epilepsy, under hospital control, they might reach a level of 3 or even 5 mmol/L—but this would take incredible levels of care as to the proteins and fats the patient was given in addition to limiting or eliminating carbs from the diet.

When someone's pancreas fails to work and ketone production becomes unregulated, that persons level of ketones in the blood reaches 10 mmol/L or more— that's ketoacidosis. That's why Type 1 diabetics need to take insulin—their pancreas doesn't produce insulin, so they need to inject it. Eating a low-carb diet will not put you into ketoacidosis.

Recently, the diet industry has latched on to what had been a term reserved for the medical community—ketogenic. You can find lots of books about ketogenic diets or ketogenic cookbooks. For the most part, all these books targeted at people who aren't doctors and are often just promoting specific low-carb/high-fat diets and recipes. And they are a great source for meal tips and planning.

But getting back to ketones…

You can think of ketones as fat energy—just like glucose is carbohydrate energy.

Our bodies run very well on ketones. I see ketones as the body's preferred fuel because molecule for molecule, ketones produce more energy than glucose. Some say the body prefers glucose because it uses glucose first. But, as I mention earlier in the book, I think the body uses glucose first because it's so easy to get too much glucose in the blood, so the body tries to get rid of it before it causes damage, even if it's not such a great fuel.

Where insulin works to store fat, a hormone called glucagon works to burn fat—both directly, and by promoting the production of ketone bodies which, in turn, supply our cells with the energy they need to function (instead of getting the energy from glucose). When insulin is high, glucagon is kept from doing its job. For glucagon to promote the creation of ketones from fat, insulin must be low. When we eat a lot of carbs our insulin level rises to deal with the glucose in the blood, and the production of ketones stops.

When insulin levels are low enough, our body recognizes our stored fat as a vast energy source. Even a lean person has enough body fat to live three or so weeks without eating anything. When burning ketones, the body does NOT slow down its metabolism when fasting. Some studies even show metabolism _rises_ when in ketosis—so you can feel more energetic[35]. When in ketosis, you can lose weight without the body trying to get you to gain it back like it does when you eat less.

Your body can only store a relatively small amount of glucose as glucose or glycogen. If the body is used to running on glucose, it will act as if glucose is the only source of energy for the body. That means if the supply of glucose is reduced (like between meals) or there is an increased demand for energy during the day (you go to the gym) the body adjusts. The first adjustment is to make us hungry, so we take in more glucose. If that doesn't work, the system slows us down so the rest of the day we don't move so much (we feel tired).

When the body gets used to burning ketones from stored fat, it can tell how much stored energy we have. It won't need to slow you down until you have very little stored fat—nearly skin and bones. At my heaviest, I was 365 pounds (166 kg). As of now, I've lost about 176 pounds (80 kg). At about 3500 calories per pound (455 grams), that's over half a million calories! At 2165 calories per day, I could have, theoretically, lived for 234 days without eating. The record for fasting is 382 days by a man in Scotland (he did take vitamin supplements). He lost 276 pounds (125 kg) in the process.

When an insulin-normal person goes to sleep (without a bedtime snack) they will spend at least part of the night in ketosis. They will come out of ketosis when they eat carbs or protein (and even likely if they eat fat, because most fat has some protein in with it).

When a person with high enough resting insulin levels goes to sleep, they might not go into ketosis because their insulin levels, even without eating, prevent glucagon from doing its job. They will often wake up very hungry in the morning—or even wake up during the night from being so hungry and raid the fridge.

Eating a low-carb/high-fat diet can help lower an insulin resistant person's resting insulin level to allow them to enter ketosis at night. Fasting acts to allow ketosis (fat burning) to take place for a longer period of time and get the body used to using both glucose and body fat for energy (it will be able to use dietary fat for energy as well).

It can take a few weeks of eating a LCHF diet to get what's called "fat adapted." Your body needs to get used to switching fuels. Also, carbs—especially sugar—can be addicting. We all know people addicted to chips or pretzels or pizza or a certain cereal or brand of cookies. You don't usually hear people saying they are addicted to steak or porkchops.

As I mentioned earlier in the book, you might go through carb-withdrawal switching to a LCHF diet—and you might experience some of these symptoms if you try an extended fast. Common symptoms include feeling weak or tired or even nauseous. You could get constipation or diarrhea. And you could get that dizzy feeling if you stand up too quickly. But like the withdrawal symptoms from any addiction, I think they are worth going through for the sake of your health.

Appendix DAIRY

Dairy is a word that seems to bring out the rabid, food-police in some people. Just say, "dairy" and watch them launch into a spiel about how bad it is, that humans are the only animal that drinks milk from another species (completely not true), and that no other adult/mature animal drinks milk (also not true—give your cat some half-n-half, or cheese, and watch how greedily they go after it).

But some people can't handle dairy products. They are lactose intolerant or have other issues. For everyone else: are dairy products good for us? Do the benefits outweigh the negatives? A quick search on the health benefits of dairy brings up a slew of articles, from mainstream health/medical groups, generally, saying that dairy is a good source of protein, calcium, and vitamin D, but it might be bad for us because of the saturated fats. There are also a slew of articles saying we don't need it and it's detrimental. So, who do we believe and why should we believe them?

Since we really aren't concerned about saturated fat, and somewhat skeptical of anyone including that in their nutritional stance or argument, we'll have to dig a bit deeper into newer, quality research.

It seems that tolerance of lactose, the sugar found in milk, is relatively new; only dating back less than 7,500 years and only in certain populations. The gene mutation which allowed lifelong consumption of milk, most likely, started in central Europe and central Balkans among the livestock raising people. Other groups, say, the Chinese, Mongolians, Native Americans, various African groups, remain lactose intolerant and become ill when drinking milk.

The rate of lactose intolerance is around 10% for Europeans, up to 95% for some Asian and African groups, and, worldwide, estimated to average 65%. If you have gas, bloating, intestinal cramps, and diarrhea after drinking milk, it's pretty safe to say you are lactose intolerant.

Obviously, for many people, drinking milk is a bad idea. But what about people that are lactose **tolerant**? Is milk nutritious? Are there too many sugars?

One cup of whole milk provides 149 calories, 8 grams of protein, 12 grams of carbohydrate (all of which are sugar), 8 grams of total fat and 5 grams of saturated fat. Carbs, protein, and fat vary depending on whether the milk is whole, 2%, 1% or skim. The lower the fat percentage, the higher the carbs. The higher the fat percentage, the lower the carbs (this would be comparing the same volume of low fat or high fat dairy product. One cup of heavy cream has 7 grams of carbs and 88 grams total fat. One cup of skim milk has 13 grams of carbs and zero grams of fat). So, if you are counting carbs, or restricting them, half and half and heavy cream are a better trade-off if you are cooking with milk or adding it to your coffee.

One cup of lactose-free milk (2 percent low fat) provides 122 calories, 8 grams of protein, 12 grams of carbohydrate (all of which are sugar), 3 grams of saturated fat and 5 grams of total fat.

There are 183 milligrams of omega-3 fatty acids per cup of whole milk and 293 milligrams of omega-6 fatty acids.

Milk is a very good source of calcium, phosphorus, vitamin D, riboflavin, and vitamin B12. It is also a good source of selenium, potassium, pantothenic acid, thiamin, and zinc.

Looking at the big picture I prefer to get my protein, fats, and micro-nutrients from sources other than milk. That said, I use half and half in my coffee, but the enjoyment I get from it far outweigh the few carbs.

Cheeses and Whey:

Cheeses, and yogurt, have far less lactose in them than milk. Many people that are lactose intolerant can safely eat them without discomfort. Your body will tell you if you shouldn't eat them! For the most part cheeses are low in carbs. The longer a cheese is aged, the lower the carbs, because the bacteria that is making the cheese is consuming the milk sugars. Also, the lower the moisture, the higher the protein.

Cottage cheese, ricotta, and cream cheese, while still being relatively low in carbs, per ounce, but also lower in protein, may not be a good choice because we tend to eat them in very large amounts. When I eat them, I try to be aware of how much I'm taking in.

Here is a handy listing originally sourced from the USDA Food Composition Databases and found at: <u>THE FULL BREAKDOWN OF CARBS IN CHEESE</u>.

Here are a few links to give you a greater understanding of milk consumption and its history:

<u>Why humans have evolved to drink milk</u>
<u>Milk Drinking Started Around 7,500 Years Ago In Central Europe</u>

Appendix VITAMINS & MINERALS

<u>Vitamin A</u> – is fat soluble (you need to consume it with fat for it to get into your system). It is good for vision, skin, the immune system, reproduction, it is a potent antioxidant fighting against cell damage, and it helps the heart, lungs, and kidneys to function properly. Beta carotene, the precursor to Vitamin A is found in orange foods such as carrots, sweet potato, and cantaloupe, as well as: dark, leafy greens, broccoli, eggs, and yellow vegetables. Because it is fat soluble, and often found bound up in fibrous foods, eating these foods with fats greatly increases its bioavailability. See the <u>Vitamin A Fact Sheet</u> (The National Institutes of Health – Office of Dietary Supplements) for more info on Vitamin A.

<u>Vitamin B Group</u> – Energy production, immune function and iron absorption. This crucial group of nutrients can be found in whole unprocessed foods, specifically whole grains, potatoes, bananas, lentils, chili peppers, beans, yeast and molasses.

There are eight types of vitamin B:
- Thiamin (B1) Essential for glucose metabolism, and it plays a key role in nerve, muscle, and heart function.
- Riboflavin Necessary for normal cell growth and function.
- Niacin Used by your body to turn food into energy.
- Pantothenic acid Animals require pantothenic acid in order to synthesize coenzyme-A (CoA), as well as to synthesize and metabolize proteins, carbohydrates, and fats.
- Biotin Your body needs biotin to help convert certain nutrients into energy. It also plays an important role in the health of your hair, skin, and nails.
- Vitamin B6 (pyridoxine) Its active form, pyridoxal 5'-phosphate, serves as a coenzyme in some 100 enzyme reactions in amino acid, glucose, and lipid metabolism.
- Folate (see below)
- Vitamin B12 (cyanocobalamin) A water-soluble vitamin involved in the metabolism of every cell of the human body: it is a cofactor in DNA

- synthesis, and in both fatty acid and amino acid metabolism. It is particularly important in the normal functioning of the nervous system via its role in the synthesis of myelin, and in the maturation of developing red blood cells in the bone marrow.

<u>Vitamin C</u> – (ascorbic acid and ascorbate) helps to repair tissues, is involved in the production of certain neurotransmitters, strengthens blood vessels, helps give skin its elasticity, is an antioxidant, and facilitates iron absorption.

"Vitamin C deficiency is rare in the United States and Canada. People who get little or no vitamin C (below about 10 mg per day) for many weeks can get scurvy. Scurvy causes fatigue, inflammation of the gums, small red or purple spots on the skin, joint pain, poor wound healing, and corkscrew hairs." <u>(NIH)</u> Vitamin C is the only essential vitamin not found in useful amounts in cooked animal products (excluding organ meats). Low amounts can be found in raw fish, meat, roe, etc. Better sources of Vitamin C include: citrus fruit, some leafy greens, broccoli, kale, Brussel sprouts, peppers, and parsley.

<u>Vitamin D (D3 and D2)</u> – is not really a vitamin. It is a secosteroid / pre-hormone. It is a multi-functional molecule necessary for calcium and energy metabolism and so much more. Vitamin D deficiency is strongly associated with diabetes, obesity, atherosclerosis, blood disorders, multiple sclerosis, thyroid disorders, autoimmune disorders (including asthmas), inflammation, and more. Vitamin D receptors are in almost all the cells in the human body.

It is almost impossible to emphasize the importance of Vitamin D too strongly. It is a metabolite that has been with us since the very beginning of our development as a species. In fact, it was Vitamin D that allowed us to evolve out of the sea. In randomized controlled trials, doses of 2,000 iu (international units) of Vitamin D3 have been shown to decrease hypertension, and 4,000 iu have shown a 63% reduction in respiratory infection.

We used to get Vitamin D from the sun (UVB)—upwards of 12,000 iu from 30 minutes of strong sunlight. But since the advent of the Industrial Revolution, when we started spending most of our time working indoors, our sun exposure, and levels of Vitamin D, have plummeted. Now we get more of it from (supplemented) foods and supplements.

Broadly speaking, sunlight has always been the largest source of Vitamin, but sunscreens block UVB, and we get so little sun, it's not a good source for most people. Some processed foods are supplemented with Vitamin D, but, unless you're eating organ meats, marrow, fatty fish, egg yolks, mushrooms, etc. you might not be getting an adequate amount.

The RDA for Vitamin D is 400 to 800 iu per day (NIH). Many studies and reputable researchers argue that this is not near enough. The U.S. National Academy of Medicine suggests that a daily intake up to 4,000 IU of vitamin D per day is safe for most people.

For a fascinating, and rigorous, presentation on Vitamin D, please go to:

D is for Debacle - The Crucial Story of Vitamin D and Human Health.

(Also see: Vitamin K)

Vitamin E – blood circulation, and protection from free radicals. Our favorite Vitamin E-rich food is the mighty almond. You can also fill up on other nuts, sunflower seeds and tomatoes to reap the benefits.

Vitamin K – is a family of fat-soluble vitamins that are instrumental in blood coagulation and appears to work synergistically with Vitamin D for proper bone mineralization. It also appears to play a role in directing calcium to the bones and away from the arteries. Food sources high in Vitamin K include: Natto (MK-7 form), Brussel sprouts, kale, broccoli, spinach, turnip and collard greens.

Vitamin K1 is found in leafy, green vegetables. Vitamin K2 (MK-4) is found in eggs, meat, and liver. Vitamin K2 (MK-7) is found in fermented foods. Vitamin K1 is responsible for regulating blood clotting. Vitamin K2 activates Vitamins A and D and contributes to bone, heart, and artery health.

Vitamin K - Fact Sheet for Health Professionals (NIH)
The Synergistic Interplay between Vitamins D and K for Bone and Cardiovascular Health: A Narrative Review (NCBI)
Comparison of MK-4 and MK-7 bioavailability in healthy women (NCBI)
Vitamin K2: Are You Consuming Enough?

Calcium – healthy teeth and bones, nerve signaling, muscle contractions, and maintaining heart rhythm. Deficiencies in calcium include numbness/tingling in the digits, tiredness, heart arrhythmia, muscle cramps, and, in some cases, convulsions.

While dietary calcium is inversely related to heart disease, calcium supplements, in studies, shows the opposite. It seems that, about eight hours after taking a calcium supplement, it can raise your blood pressure and your blood coagulates more (blood platelet activation).

Yogurt, cheese and milk, tofu, leafy greens, broccoli, sardines, and beans/lentils are good sources of calcium. Here is a <u>list</u>, from the International Osteoporosis Foundation, of calcium in common foods.

<u>Choline</u> – is neither vitamin nor mineral. It is a water-soluble compound that is a precursor needed to make acetylcholine. The body makes a small amount of it, but it is an essential nutrient you get from food, that is important for DNA synthesis, nerve and muscle function, memory, cell structure development, cell messaging, and a deficiency, while rare, can lead to fatty liver.

Beef liver, chicken liver, eggs, fresh cod, salmon, cauliflower, broccoli, and nuts are high in choline.

<u>Choline - Fact Sheet for Health Professionals</u> (NIH)

<u>Chromium</u> – is a trace mineral, a metallic element, needed, by the body, in very small amounts. It is thought to be beneficial to insulin sensitivity, protein synthesis, carb and fat metabolism. Deficiencies are rare and exactly how much is needed is unclear.

<u>Co-Q10</u> – Ubiquinol is a fat-soluble enzyme that is part of the cellular energy production pathway. It is often taken for heart health and is thought to be a potent antioxidant. Low levels of Co-Q10 are associated with heart failure, chest pain, and high blood pressure. Co-Q10 might also be helpful in preventing tissue damage from surgery, might ease diabetic neuropathy, and has shown some effect on migraines. It is not approved, in the U.S., for medical treatment. Deficiencies are rare and good sources are cold-water fish (tuna, salmon, mackerel, and sardines), vegetable oils, and meats. See <u>Coenzyme Q10</u> (NIH) for more info.

<u>Folic Acid / Folate / Vitamin B9</u> – Folic acid is a synthetic compound that is then converted into methyl folate. Methyl folate is the actual vitamin used in the body. The enzyme that converts folic acid into methyl folate, dihydrofolate reductase, works very well in lab rats, but very poorly in humans. This leaves folic acid hanging around in the body, and it is methyl folate that is bioactive; folic acid is, essentially, inert, but the methyl folate receptors prefer folic acid.

That means the excess folic acid, left over from inefficient conversion to methyl folate, binds up the methyl folate receptors thereby blocking the use of methyl folate. It is much better to get your folate from leafy greens, liver, or, if using a supplement, it should be listed as: 5-methyltetrahydrofolate, 5-MTHF, methyl THF, or methyl folate.

Methyl folate is effective in reducing headaches, pain, cardiovascular disease risk and thrombosis, preeclampsia, periodontal disease, increases nitric oxide, and is needed to help form healthy cells. It is also a precursor to the production of serotonin, norepinephrine, and dopamine. Proper levels of folate are strongly associated with a reduction in neural tube defects in newborns.

Foods high in folate include: citrus fruits, legumes, asparagus, broccoli, Brussel sprouts, eggs, leafy greens, beets, liver, nuts/seeds, bananas, and avocado.

Iron – is an important component of hemoglobin. Hemoglobin is the part of the red blood cell that transports oxygen throughout the body. Low iron is the most common nutritional deficiency in the U.S. If you don't have enough iron, you can't make enough red blood cells and the condition, with symptoms including exhaustion, weakness, shortness of breath, and fast heartbeat, is called "iron deficiency anemia". Iron is also important for healthy cells, skin, hair, and nails.

Women have a higher daily need for iron than men, but kidney failure, certain gastro-intestinal disorders (that inhibit the absorption of iron), excessive use of antacids, and intense exercise (through the destruction of red blood cells) can cause a higher need for iron.

Good sources are: clams, oysters, organ meats, soybeans, pumpkin seeds, beans, lentils, and spinach.

Magnesium – This mineral plays an important role in muscle contractions. It is also a natural muscle relaxant and can help smooth muscles, including your intestines. It also helps another essential vitamin, calcium, to absorb. It can be found in natural sources such as spinach and other leafy greens. It is also found in almonds and beans.

Omega-3 – It is thought that humans evolved on a diet consisting of a 1 to 1 ratio of Omega-3 fatty acids to Omega-6 fatty acids. The standard Western diet is about 1 to 15, so we are very deficient in Omega-3's. A great deal of our (excessive) Omega-6's come from vegetable oils and processed foods. Closing down the ratio, getting closer to 1:1, reduces the incidence of cardiovascular disease, cancer, and assorted inflammatory and autoimmune diseases (diseases that proliferate with high Omega-6 – low Omega-3).

Good sources of Omega-3:
- Fish and other seafood (especially cold-water fatty fish, such as salmon, mackerel, tuna, herring, and sardines)
- Nuts and seeds (such as flaxseed, chia seeds, and walnuts)
- Plant oils (such as flaxseed oil, soybean oil, and canola oil)
- <u>Fortified</u> foods (such as certain brands of eggs, yogurt, juices, milk, soy beverages

Please see: <u>Omega-3 Fatty Acids -Fact Sheet for Consumers</u> for more information.

<u>Potassium</u> – is a mineral and an electrolyte. It helps your muscles work, including the muscles that control your heartbeat and breathing. Your body uses the potassium it needs. The extra potassium that your body does not need is removed from your blood by your kidneys.

Potassium plays a role in keeping your body well-hydrated. In fact, it is used in almost all of the body's functions, including: proper kidney and heart function, muscle contraction, nerve transmission, and bone health.

Potassium deficiency (Hypokalemia): There are many different reasons you could have low potassium levels. It may be because too much potassium is leaving through your digestive tract. It's usually a symptom of another problem. Most commonly, you get hypokalemia when:
- You vomit a lot
- You have diarrhea
- Your kidneys or adrenal glands don't work well
- You take medication that makes you pee (water pills or diuretics)

It's possible, but rare, to get hypokalemia from having too little potassium in your diet. Other things sometimes cause it, too, like:
- Drinking too much alcohol
- Sweating a lot
- Folic acid deficiency

- Certain antibiotics
- Laxatives taken over a long period of time
- Certain types of tobacco
- Some asthma medications
- Low magnesium

Symptoms of low potassium include: weakness/fatigue, muscle cramping or twitching, constipation, and irregular heartbeat. Severe hypokalemia is rare in healthy people with normal kidney function.

Good sources of potassium include: fruits (such as dried apricots, prunes, raisins, orange juice, and bananas), vegetables (acorn squash, potatoes, spinach, tomatoes, and broccoli, lentils, kidney beans, soybeans, and nuts), milk and yogurt, meats, poultry, and fish.

Please follow this link: <u>Potassium - Fact Sheet for Consumers</u> to learn more.

<u>Zinc</u> – a mineral, is called an "essential trace element" because very small amounts of zinc are necessary for human health. Since our bodies don't store excess zinc, it must be consumed on a regular basis.

Zinc supports the immune system, cell division, the sense of taste and smell, wound healing, and it might slow the progression of age-related macular degeneration. It plays a role in growth, fertility, libido, and, when taken immediately at the onset of a cold, might reduce duration and symptoms.

Intranasal sprays are associated with loss of smell. Sometimes permanently.
Too much zinc can lead to: nausea, vomiting, abdominal cramps, loss of appetite, apathy, diarrhea, and headaches.

Good sources of zinc include: oysters, beef, chicken, tofu, pork, nuts, lentils, yogurt, oatmeal, and mushrooms.
<u>Zinc - Fact Sheet for Health Professionals</u> (NIH)

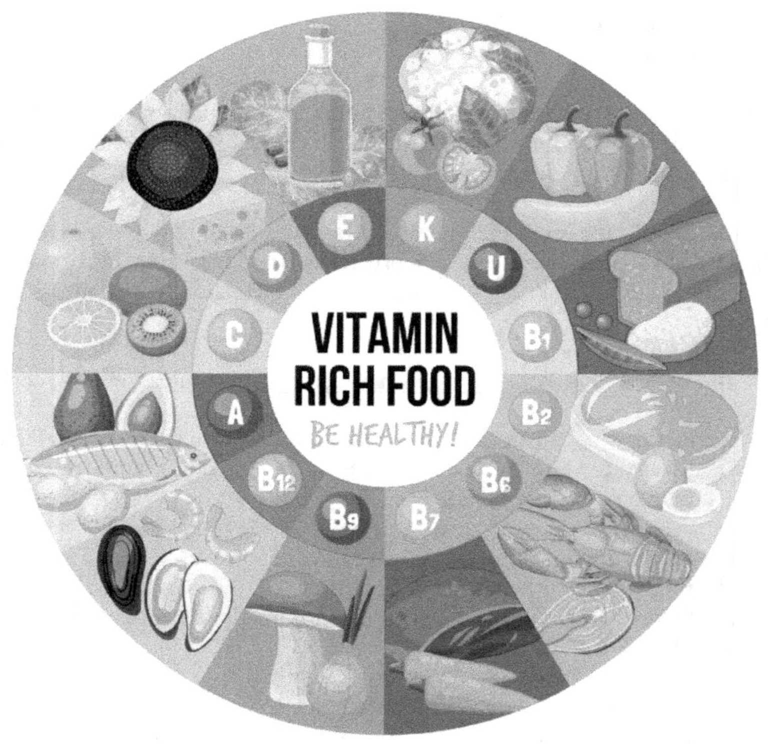

Hopefully, you've made it through all of that without getting horribly bored and only slightly confused. You'll note that I didn't list any of the RDA levels and that is for some very good reasons: in a nutshell, everyone is different. Short, tall, young, old, healthy, unhealthy, different ethnic and genetic backgrounds, different levels, and types, of activities, etc. play a role in how much you need of which vitamin and mineral.

Trying to pin down how much you need, with any precision, and how much you are getting from your food and/or supplements, is a very difficult, if not impractical, task.

Then throw in the synergistic, or antagonistic, effect among the various vitamins and minerals, and you are certain to be confused.

Which brings up a very interesting question: should we take vitamin and mineral supplements? The short answer is: we really don't know. Some people, doctors and nutritionists among them, say we should. Others say we don't need to.

If you are eating a diet of meats and vegetables, and don't have any health issues, you might be getting enough of all the things you need and not too much (which can be toxic).

It really is best to have a blood panel done through your doctor and see if you are deficient in anything or if anything looks out of whack.

That said, there are some very common deficiencies: (heme) iron, calcium, Vitamin D, magnesium, iodine, Vitamin B12, Vitamin A, and folate.

These articles are worth reading, if only to give you something to think about:
7 Nutrient Deficiencies That Are Incredibly Common
Iron, Folate, and Other Essential Vitamins You're Not Getting Enough of (and Really Should)
Vitamins and Minerals Are You Getting What You Need?

This presentation is definitely worth watching:
Why You Shouldn't RELY on Vitamin and Mineral Supplements

References

1. Source: Data for 1971-2014: Fryar, C. D., Carroll, M. D., & Ogden, C. L. (2016). Prevalence of overweight and obesity among children and adolescents aged 2-19 years: United States, 1963-1965 through 2013-2014. Hyattsville, MD: U.S. Department of Health and Human Services, Centers for Disease Control and Prevention, National Center for Health Statistics. Retrieved from https://www.cdc.gov/nchs/data/hestat/obesity_child_13_14/obesity_child_13_14.pdf. Data for 2015-2016: Hales, C. M., Carroll, M. D., Fryar, C. D., & Ogden, C. L. (2017). Prevalence of obesity among adults and youth: United States, 2015-2016 (NSCH Data Brief No. 288). Hyattsville, MD: U.S. Department of Health and Human Services, Centers for Disease Control and Prevention, National Center for Health Statistics. Retrieved from https://www.cdc.gov/nchs/products/databriefs/db288.htm

2. Dietary Guidelines for Americans, Eighth Edition, 2015 - 2020 https://www.dietaryguidelines.gov/sites/default/files/2019-05/2015-2020_Dietary_Guidelines.pdf

3. Lehninger, A., Nelson, D. and Cox, M. Principles of Biochemistry

4. Prevention of coronary and stroke events with atorvastatin in hypertensive patients who have average or lower-than-average cholesterol concentrations, in Anglo-Scandinavian Cardiac Outcomes Trial—Lipid Lowering Arm: a multicenter randomized controlled trial. The Lancet, Volume 361, April 2003.

5. Stampfer, M. J.; Willett, W. C.; Colditz, G. A.; Rosner, B.; Speizer, F. E.; Hennekens, C. H. (1985-10-24). "A prospective study of postmenopausal estrogen therapy and coronary heart disease". *The New England Journal of Medicine*. **313** (17): 1044–1049.

6. https://medicalxpress.com/news/2018-11-high-protein-diet-affect-kidney-function.html

7. Weight Loss with a Low-Carbohydrate, Mediterranean, or Low-Fat Diet, Iris Shai, R.D., Ph.D., Dan Schwarzfuchs, M.D., Yaakov Henkin, M.D., Danit R. Shahar, R.D., Ph.D., Shula Witkow, R.D., M.P.H., Ilana Greenberg, R.D., M.P.H., Rachel Golan, R.D., M.P.H., Drora Fraser, Ph.D., Arkady Bolotin, Ph.D., Hilel Vardi, M.Sc., Osnat Tangi-Rozental, B.A., Rachel Zuk-Ramot,

R.N., et al., July 17, 2008, New England Journal of Medicine, 2008; 359:229-241, DOI: 10.1056/NEJMoa0708681.

8. Effectiveness and Safety of a Novel Care Model for the Management of Type 2 Diabetes at 1 Year: An Open-Label, Non-Randomized, Controlled Study, Sarah J. Hallberg, Amy L. McKenzie, Paul T. Williams, Nasir H. Bhanpuri, Anne L. Peters, Wayne W. Campbell, Tamara L. Hazbun, Brittanie M. Volk, James P. McCarter, Stephen D. Phinney, and Jeff S. Volek, Diabetes Therory, 2018 Apr; 9(2): 583–612.

9. www.publichealthcollaboration.org

10. https://www.cdc.gov/media/releases/2017/p0718-diabetes-report.html

11. Anton, SD et al. Effects of Stevia, Aspartame, and Sucrose on Food Intake, Satiety, and Postprandial Glucose and Insulin Levels. Appetite. 2010, August; 55(1):37-43

12. Dokken, BB and Tsao, T-S, The Physiology of Body Weight Regulation: Are We Too Efficient for Our Own Good? Diabetes Spectrum Vol 20, Number 3: 166-170, 2007

13. Morton GJ, Cummings DE, Baskin DG, Barsh GS, Schwartz MW: Central nervous system control of food intake and body weight. *Nature* 443:289–295, 2006

14. Rosenbaum M, Leibel RL: The physiology of body weight regulation: relevance to the etiology of obesity in children. *Pediatrics* 101:525–539, 1998

15. Leibel RL, Rosenbaum M, Hirsch J: Changes in energy expenditure resulting from altered body weight. *New England Journal of Medicine* 332:621–628, 1995

16. Wadden TA: Treatment of obesity by moderate and severe caloric restriction: results of clinical research trials. *Annals of Internal Medicine* 119:688–693, 1993

17. Keesey RE, Powley TL: The regulation of body weight. *Annual Review of Psychology* 37:109–133, 1986

18. Sims EA, Danforth E Jr, Horton ES, Bray GA, Glennon JA, Salans LB. Endocrine and metabolic effects of experimental obesity in man. Recent Progress in Hormone Research, 1973;29:457-96

19. Fung J. The Obesity Code, Scribe Publications, London, UK, 2016.

20. Zihlman, A and Bolter, D. Body composition in Pan paniscus compared with Homo sapiens has implications for changes during human evolution, Proceedings of the National Academy of Sciences, June, 2015.

21. Griffin, B. et al, Role of plasma triglyceride in the regulation of plasma low density lipoprotein (LDL) subfractions: relative contribution of small, dense

LDL to coronary heart disease risk, Atherosclerosis, Volume 106, Issue 2, April 1994, Pages 241-253

22. Benton, D and Young, H: Reducing Calorie Intake May Not Help You Lose Body Weight, Perspectives on Psychological Science, 2017 Sep; 12(5): 703–714.

23. Santos FL, Esteves SS, da Costa Pereira A, Yancy WS Jr, Nunes JP. Systematic review and meta-analysis of clinical trials of the effects of low carbohydrate diets on cardiovascular risk factors. Obesity Review. 2012 Nov;13(11):1048-66.

24. Dashti, H. et al. Long-term effects of ketogenic diet in obese subjects with high cholesterol. Molecular and Cellular Biochemistry 286: 1-6, 2006.

25. Harlan, W et al. Familial hypercholesterolemia: a genetic and metabolic study. Medicine, 1966, Vol 45, No 2.

26. Risk of fatal coronary heart disease in familial hypercholesterolaemia. Scientific Steering Committee on behalf of the Simon Broome Register Group. British Journal of Medicine, Volume 303, October 1991.

27. Schatz, I. et al. Cholesterol and all-cause mortality in elderly people from the Honolulu Heart Study: a cohort study. Lancet, 2001; 358: 351 – 355.

28. Ludwig, DS et al. High glycemic index foods, overeating, and obesity. Pediatrics, 1999 Mar;103(3): E26.

29. Ebbeling, CB et al. Effects of dietary composition on energy expenditure during weight-loss maintenance. Journal of the American Medical Association, 2012 Jun 27;307(24):2627-34.

30. Thomas, DE, Elliot, EJ and Baur, L. Low glycaemic index or low glycaemic load diets for overweight and obesity. Cochrane Database Systematic Review, 2007 Jul 18;(3):CD005105.

31. Ebbeling, CB et al. Effects of a low carbohydrate diet on energy expenditure during weight loss maintenance: randomized trial. British Medical Journal, 2018;363.

32. Juntenen, K et al. Postprandial glucose, insulin, and incretin responses to grain products in healthy subjects. American Journal of Clinical Nutrition, 2002; 75 (2): 254 – 262.

33. Banting, W. Letter on Corpulence, 1863, Pantianos Classics.

34. Swift, DL et al. The Role of Exercise and Physical Activity in Weight Loss and Maintenance. Progress in Cardiovascular Diseases. 2014 Jan-Feb; 56(4): 441–447.

35. Drenick, EJ et al. Energy expenditure in fasting obese men. The Journal of Laboratory and Clinical Medicine. March 1973: Volume 81, Issue 3, Pages 421–430.

36. Taken from the American Grassfed Association website: www.americangrassfed.org
37. Antibiotics in Your Food: Should You be Concerned? From Healthline.com
38. See www.webmd.com for more details
39. See www.epa.gov for more details
40. Tilapia Fish: Benefits and Dangers, taken from Healthline.com
41. Mythbusting 101: Organic Farming > Conventional Agriculture. Taken from blogs.scientificamerican.com
42. Food Labels: Definition of Natural & Organic, from livescience.com
43. The 'uncured' bacon illusion: It's actually cured, and it's not better for you, from the Washington Post (online)
44. Dirt Poor: Have Fruits and Vegetables Become Less Nutritious? From scientificamerican.com
45. The Best Oils for Cooking, and Which to Avoid, from BonAppetit.com
46. Venkata, RP and Subramanyam R. Evaluation of the deleterious health effects of consumption of repeatedly heated vegetable oil. Toxicology Reports, 2016; 3: 636–643.
47. PUFA: What is it and Why Should it Be Avoided? From butterbeliever.com

Suggested Reading List

- The Obesity Code, by Jason Fung
- The Complete Guide to Fasting, by Jason Fung with Jimmy Moore
- The Case Against Sugar, by Gary Taubes
- Good Calories, Bad Calories, by Gary Taubes
- Why We Get Fat, by Gary Taubes
- The Big Fat Surprise, by Nina Teicholz
- The Real Meal Revolution, by Tim Noakes, Junno Proudfoot and Sally-Ann Creed
- Advanced Nutrition and Human Metabolism 7th Edition, by Sareen S. Gropper, Jack L. Smith and Timothy P. Carr

Part 4: LCHF IN THE KITCHEN

I've wrestled with what to share in this section. It isn't a cookbook, nor does it have a hundred recipes (but check the web site, I'll be putting recipes there). It isn't meant to dive into all the techniques, large and small, that go into making a meal. It is, instead, a brief overview of what I eat that is LCHF, some basic, foundational skills that are in constant use, and a way of thinking about food and ingredients. –Evan

In my mind, to successfully move to a new way of eating, you must always ask:
1. Is it good for me?
2. Do I like it?
3. Will I eat it?

You need to answer yes to these three questions, otherwise you will revert back to unhealthy foods.

So, approach this new way of eating with an open mind. Try different foods and food combinations. Experiment. The goal is to identify foods that are good for you, that you like and that you will eat. If you only eat the meals you are used to—minus the carbs—you will likely revert back to eating the carbs as well because something will seem "missing" from your meals.

Steven's Side Note: I found that once I embraced the idea that saturated fat was good for me, a lot of foods became regulars on my menu, like pork and beef ribs and greasy burgers (no bun). But I also tried foods I'd never eaten before like bone broth, boiled, fatty cuts of meat, even things like beef tongue and beef heart (if you weren't told what they were, you'd think they were some sort of sliced lunchmeat). I've even tried cow cheek, pig cheek (both highly recommended) and cow brain (glad I tried it— just to say I did it—but I don't recommend it). Living in northern Italy, it's easier to sample these things as they are traditional menu items. But as Evan says, experiment and keep an open mind!

Tools of the Trade

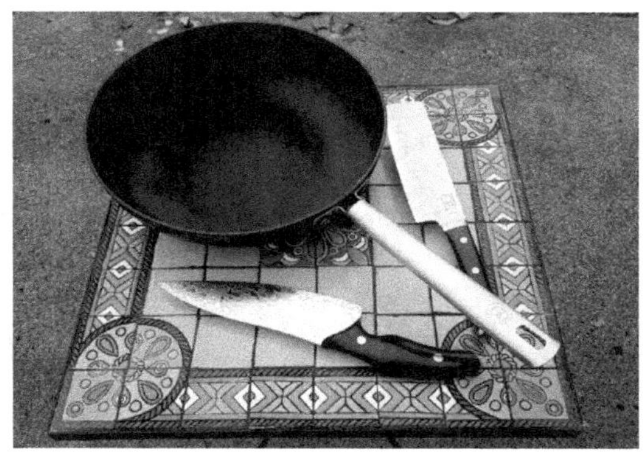

The pan in the picture is a 12-inch, Analon professional, hard anodized, nonstick, long-handled wok. I purchased it at least 15 years ago. This thing gets used all the time and has held up extremely well. It wasn't overly expensive.

The quality of your pots and pans will make a huge difference in performance and will add to the enjoyment of cooking. Little things, like a handle that doesn't get hot and is easy to grip, the curve of the walls, the general balance, even heating (no hot spots), and the feel of solid construction, when you use a pan every day, or nearly every day, become big issues when those attributes are wrong or flawed.

Price is a consideration when purchasing pots and pans, but that doesn't mean you have to buy the most expensive pieces to get the best quality. There are plenty of high-priced items in the world that aren't, necessarily, the highest quality. In fact, in the middle range, for consumer prices, you can get great pieces at an affordable price.

I've been very impressed with Calphalon and Analon hard anodized, nonstick pieces. You can get a 10-inch skillet for around $50.00. A small, but full set of pots and pans from Calphalon (on Amazon) is $170.00 which will more than adequately meet your needs. The set includes:

- 8" Fry Pan

- 10" Fry Pan

- 2.5 qt. Saucepan with Cover + No Boil-Over Insert

- 3 qt. Sauté Pan with Cover

- 6 qt. Stock Pot with Cover + No Boil-Over Insert

It's a good range of sizes, shapes, and the brand is known for putting out quality, ergonomic pieces. In comparison, one of my All Clad frying pans retails for $150 and, as much as I like it, I still reach for the my Analon wok first (half of my 19 pieces are either Analon or Calphalon; in my mind, they are very comparable).

A thickness of 3.8mm to 4mm on the walls of pots and pans is substantial enough to hold up to use. Bottom thickness will vary greatly between designs and styles. The general rule of thumb is: don't buy cheap, thin pots and pans. You'll dent them, burn food, get hot spots, and be extremely disappoint. Spending an extra 30%, at this lower to middle level, really does make a big difference.

Steven's Side Note: I bought a cheap set of pots and pans after I got divorced and they made cooking very unappealing. For me, the problem was I was always burning part of whatever I was cooking; because the pots and pans were so thin, they would burn whatever was directly over the flame of the burner. I finally went to Costco with Evan and he suggested a set of Calphalon pots and pans—more pieces than the one mentioned above but without the No Boil-Over insert (because it hadn't been invented yet). It made such a difference I can't believe I managed to cook without them. I'll add to what Evan has said to say that good cookware gives you confidence in the kitchen. PS: Neither Evan nor I work for Calphalon!

You'll want to get some decent knives. Or, at least, a good chef's knife, a slicer, and a paring knife. You can buy a complete set, with or without matching steak knives, or purchase them individually. My preference leans toward German steel, like the Wüsthof Classic series, but mid to higher end Japanese knives have come a long way.

An 8-inch chef's knife is the most flexible to use. Ten inch gets a little bit unwieldy and 6-inch just doesn't have the length needed when chopping up lots of food. A Wüsthof Classic, 8-inch chef's knife should run $125.00.

In the picture above, on the right, is a cheap Nakiri blade (rectangular) that I picked up to see if I'd like that style of blade. Turns out it is quite nice, and I'll be buying a better quality one in the future (however the one I bought far exceeds my expectations for the $20.00 that I paid for it, so I'm not rushing to spend more money). Expect to pay $40 to $80 for a good quality blade, but prices can go up to $250.

A paring knife is generally useful for all sorts of things and you'll find yourself using one quite often. $30 to $50 is a reasonable price.

The other knife, in the picture above, is a limited run, Ken Onion piece designed to be ergonomically comfortable in both the holding and the movement pattern (the front of the belly and the belly itself are slightly different arcs). It works very well but retailed at a ridiculous price and the premium paid doesn't make it perform better than a Wüsthof eight inch. But it does have a cool, funky factor.

You'll want to buy knives from a reputable manufacturer that is known for their quality steel and craftsmanship. Look for knives that have a full tang (the piece of metal between the handles should extend all the way through the end) and have a full bolster (there should be a "built up" section of the blade between the handle and the working, thin part of the blade). This will fit your hand better and helps to prevent slipping.

Buy a few different sized cutting boards and add more as you go along; once you've figured out how much space you usually need for cutting. A larger cutting board means you can keep more food on it, as you are working, but you don't want one so large it's a hassle to clean and store.

Whether you buy wood or plastic, try to buy thicker cutting boards. Thin ones will warp easily or fall apart. The material is up to you and your preference. Plastic boards can be scrubbed and bleached, to get rid of particles and bacteria, but wood boards have natural antibiotic features that help to cut down on bacteria after you've cleaned them. The jury is out on which one is actually safest. Whichever you use, just do a thorough cleaning and you should be good.

Sauté, Salts, Acids, Fats

The basic things that make certain combinations of ingredients taste so good is the presence, and balance, of salt, fat, and acids. Not only do they taste good, they work together nutritionally. Many of the nutrients found in vegetables need fat, like olive oil, to be properly digested and utilized. And an acid, whether it be a vinegar or lemon juice, cuts through the fat and helps to make other flavors pop and shine.

Imagine you have some beautiful tomatoes, fresh from the garden. Dice them, pour a liberal amount of olive oil over them, sprinkle on some balsamic or red wine vinegar, and top with granules of sea salt. Simple, tasty, nutritious, low in carbs and full of beneficial nutrients.

This can be had as a substantial side dish next to meat, you can use it in a zoodle dish, or even as an accessory topping grilled chicken or a cream-based zoodle concoction. Multiple uses from a few ingredients.

And speaking of **zoodles**:

Zoodles are the low carb substitute for grain-based pasta. They are made from zucchini, or yellow (crook neck) squash using a vegetable spiralizer. These noodles are easily cooked in the microwave (I start at 90 seconds, full power, then add small amounts of time, as needed, to get them to the texture I want), then tossed into a pan with whatever other ingredients, meats and vegetables, you are using to make a "pasta dinner."

They aren't a perfect substitute for pasta, but their flavor is relatively neutral, and, after a few tries, you'll know how to make them al dente ("to the tooth" – slightly firm to the bite). You'll want to by smaller, up to medium, sized squash for this. As zucchini/yellow squash grow larger, their flesh gets increasingly water-logged and less dense.

If you already eat a lot of pasta, this can be a very good variation. Make your pasta sauce, as usual, and toss in the zoodles. Tomato sauces, which are reasonably low carb, meats, and cream sauces work just fine. If there is water in the bowl, from heating the zoodles in the microwave, just pour it off before tossing them in with the other ingredients.

Here is my zoodle maker. One smallish squash makes enough zoodles just for me.

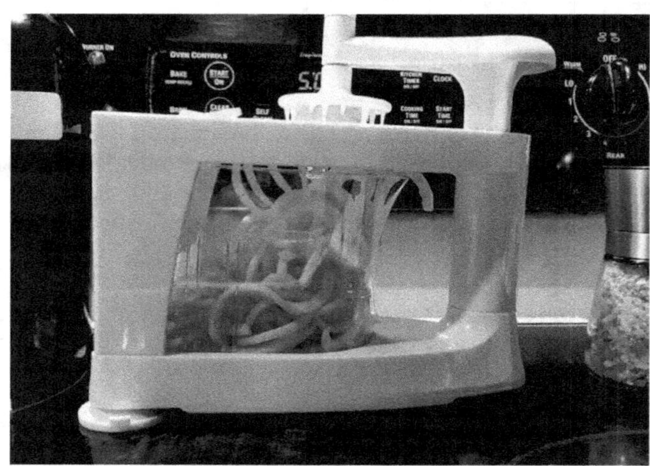

Sauté:

To cook quickly, in a small amount of oil, on high heat, uniformly sized pieces of food is called sauté. Stir-frying is cooking food over high heat, in a small amount of oil, while stirring rapidly.

So, there isn't necessarily much difference between the two except for a few things: in sauté you move the pan itself, aggressively, and flip the food, curling off the far edge and back into the pan. In stir-fry, you stir with a spatula or spoon, then as the initial ingredient cooks, you push the food upwards on the walls, leaving the center bare, then add your next ingredient(s).

When using multiple ingredients, it is best to cook the "longest to cook" food first, move the food from the center, and add the new food into the center. Because a skillet, used in sauté has a bigger, flat bottom than a wok, used in stir-fry, the food you move toward the side will tend to cook a bit faster/more than if you were using a wok.

That, for the most part, might be a distinction without a difference depending on what you are cooking and your timing when adding the ingredients.

It's worth noting the difference between a sauté pan and a skillet. You'd think a sauté pan would be preferred for, well, sautéing, but that's not always the case. A sauté pan has straight, vertical sides so, while you can stir the food easily, it is horrible for "flipping" the food and the technique of flipping is very instrumental when cooking with high heat. But, don't worry if you don't know how to do that.

A skillet has sloping, curved sides, great for flipping the food, but will have a slightly smaller, flat bottom. But not as small as a wok (some woks have flat bottoms and some having curved).

Whichever you have, or prefer to use, sauté pan, skillet, or wok (my most used pan is a high-sided wok with a long handle and a 5-inch flat bottom), some basic techniques are the same:

Because excessive heat in an empty pan can cause warpage, I thoroughly heat the pan on medium, then add olive oil, and crank the heat. You want to get the pan, and the oil, hot enough, that when you add your first ingredient, it sizzles like crazy. You'll know it's hot enough by the way the oil moves and shimmers. It physically acts different; looser, thinner, and, depending on your lighting, you'll be able to see a bit of it rising into the air; kind of like a thin vapor. Pay attention to this and you'll learn to judge by appearance when it is hot enough. Initially, if you are unsure, take a piece of food and dip it in. If it sizzles like crazy, it's ready, toss in the rest.

Generally, I'll take the longest to cook food, say broccoli, and cook it 2/3s of the way through, push it to the sides, then add whatever meat might be going in, cook that almost all the way through then, if the stove has been able to maintain the high temperature, I'll add a few glugs of white wine, and cook that down, then add a little bit of lemon juice and soy sauce, turn off the heat, move all the ingredients around a bit, then finish it with a tablespoon, or two, of butter.

You want the butter to melt, and mix in, but not separate (separation is when the oils and solid particles in butters and creams break away from each other. You'll suddenly see little blotches of oil. This is caused by too much heat, for too long, reducing too far, or adding an acid at the wrong time). So, keep the food moving just until the butter melts, then transfer to a plate.

If the stove and pan aren't able to maintain high temperature before adding white wine, I'll scooch all the food over to the sides, so the center is bare, let it get hot again, before adding the wine. I want the wine to cook down almost to nothing, but not completely gone, because I want the food to end up with more of a glaze than a soupy sauce. And there's plenty of liquid from the wine, lemon, soy sauce, combined with the butter, to do that. You don't always have to use wine, soy sauce, lemon juice, and butter. Do what tastes good to you and adjust your technique accordingly.

Use one, use two, experiment. White wine works well with butter, cream, stir-fried veggies, etc. Red wine, having a deeper, richer taste works well with beef, tomatoes (as does white wine), etc. Vinegars, in small amounts, can brighten flavors, as will a bit of hot sauce.

If your pan gets too hot, or if it's too hot for the butter, don't be afraid to move the whole thing off the heat. The slowest way to cool down a pan, even if just dropping it 10 degrees or so, is to use the knob on the stove. And you'll usually want to drop the temp quickly.

So, that's a basic cooking technique that you can use every day, as you wish. Add the longest-to-cook items first, move them to the side, then add the next, and the next. Add some wine, soy, lemon, orange juice, fish sauce, butter, whatever you like.

Let's say I was going to make a dish with thin slices of beef and thin slices of quartered tomatoes. The tomatoes might take a touch longer to cook than the beef, but I want to get a good sear of the meat. I'd toss the meat in first, let that cook for 30 seconds or so, and then add the tomatoes. Then finish appropriately.

If you are adding any dried herbs, do it right before you add the second ingredient. This way they heat up enough to release their flavors, but they won't burn. While spices and herbs are sometimes the first things heated in the pan, to "bloom" them and pull out their flavors, that is usually done when you are adding something that will suck up enough heat to stop them from frying for too long. But, if you are cooking something that needs more time, adding the dried herbs too early, can burn them and make them bitter.

Tenderizing Meat

One way to tenderize and flavor meats is to marinate beef, chicken, pork, turkey, etc. in a concoction of oil, spices, herbs, and an acid such as lemon juice or vinegar. The drawback is that letting it sit too long, depending on the size of the meat, could lead to pickling—great flavor, but mushy texture, and hard to sear.

Another way is with a wet brine (salt and water) which works ok, but is messy, needs a substantial container, and doesn't produce optimal results. It works, but not well enough.

I like to do something called "**dry brining**." To dry brine meat you cover it in a thin layer of coarse salt and let it rest in the fridge, flipping it on occasion. My understanding of how it works is that the salt pulls the moisture out of the meat, creating tiny channels in it. Then, the meat, acting like a sponge, pulls the moisture and salt deep inside. But don't worry, it won't taste overly salted. If you add some seasoning it seems to pull in that flavor, as well.

I became curious, because I eat a fair amount of pork loin, and there isn't much fat on the meat. It's very lean except for the outside rail (the covering of fat on one side of the meat). I wondered if spraying the portioned cuts, around ¾ inch thick, with olive oil, liberally salting it, then adding dried herbs, would force the oil into the meat.

I really don't know if it works that way, but I've been getting extremely moist pieces of meat, full of flavor, searing nicely in the cast iron, grilling pan, and the oil is going somewhere.

Here is what I do:

I'll take portioned, sliced pork loin, chicken breasts, and lean cuts of beef, spray a good coating of olive oil on one side, generously sprinkle with coarse salt then dried herbs, flip and repeat for the other side. I do this on top of plastic wrap. Then I wrap it up tightly and do an additional wrapping with more plastic wrap; just to make sure the liquid doesn't come out as its going through its process.

For thinner cuts of meat, like chicken breasts or pork loin, let rest in the fridge for a minimum of 40 minutes. I often leave these in the fridge for (around) 24 hours or more. Big chunks of meat should be a minimum of 24 hours and a whole turkey should sit for three days. If doing a bird, force the salt and seasonings under the skin and leave out the oil. Feel free to experiment with using oil, or going oil free, and see what works for you.

Example Meals

What follows are just a few examples of what I frequently eat. You will be able to see more examples on the web site (https://beleansecrets.com) in the coming months.

Baked, Seasoned Chicken Legs with Tomatoes

This is a very simple, but very satisfying meal. The chicken legs/drumsticks were dry brined, with herbs, and baked (see further below).

The tomatoes, fresh from the garden have been doused fairly heavily with extra virgin olive oil, a young, crude balsamic vinegar, Himalayan sea salt, and topped with sliced pepperoncini. Extra sharp cheddar cheese rounds out the plate.

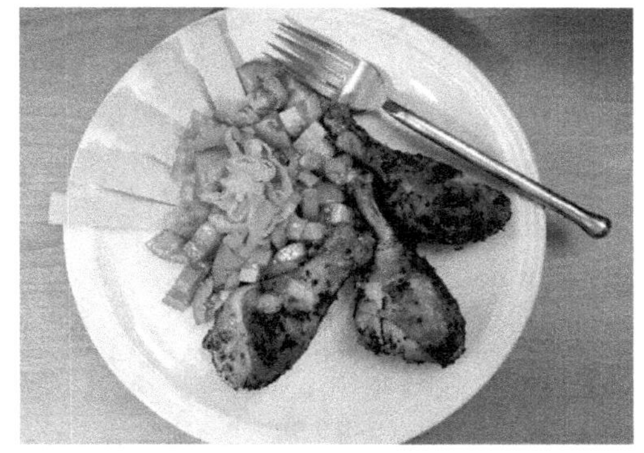

Cold Sausage and Greens

I like good, coarse bratwurst and find it works well on top of a pile of mixed, spring greens with balsamic vinegar, olive oil, sliced pepperoncini, shredded parmesan cheese, and sun dried (actually, dehydrated in the oven with Himalayan salt and crushed, red pepper) tomatoes.

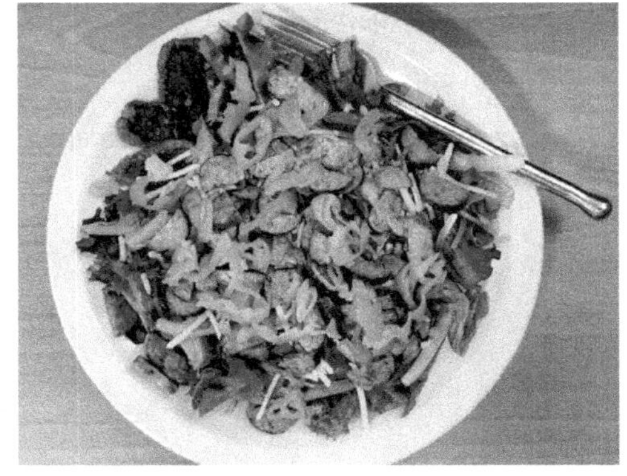

While I do enjoy a decent vinaigrette, in recent years I've been adding the oils and vinegars, separately, directly on top of my salads. Instead of having one uniform taste spread throughout, this creates different areas of flavor; little flavor bursts.

Use whatever meats, and cheeses, you want on top of a salad. Salami, ham, turkey, bacon, sliced pork, roast beef, chicken, cheddar, Swiss, blue, parmesan, and other hard cheeses … It all tastes good! And don't be afraid to use a lot of olive oil.

Ground Beef Zoodle Sauté

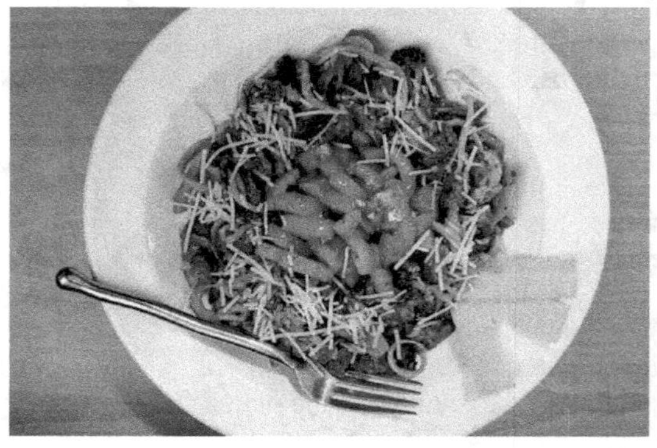

This was an interesting, little experiment in flavors. I wasn't sure if the broccoli would throw things off or not.

I started with ground beef, cooked well, scooched it up the sides of the wok, tossed in a bunch of broccoli, let that cook for a few minutes before tossing it all around in the pan, then added salt, Mexican oregano, crushed, red pepper and a few glugs of red wine. I let the liquid reduce about halfway, tossed in zoodles made with yellow squash (that I had cooked in the microwave), took the pan off the heat and add two tablespoons of salted butter.

After plating, I gave it a generous amount of shredded parmesan cheese and topped it with garden tomatoes that had been marinating for an hour in lemon juice, olive oil, salt, and a small amount of chili powder.

Surprisingly, it turned out pretty well.

Grilled Pork Loin, Broccoli, and Tomatoes

This is (slightly) thick pork loin slices that had been liberally sprayed with olive oil, covered in a pre-made, store bought BBQ rub and rested in the fridge for 18 hours. The pork was then "grilled" in a heavy, cast iron grilling pan (it has raised ridges) to medium doneness.

The broccoli was a simple stir-fry started in olive oil and 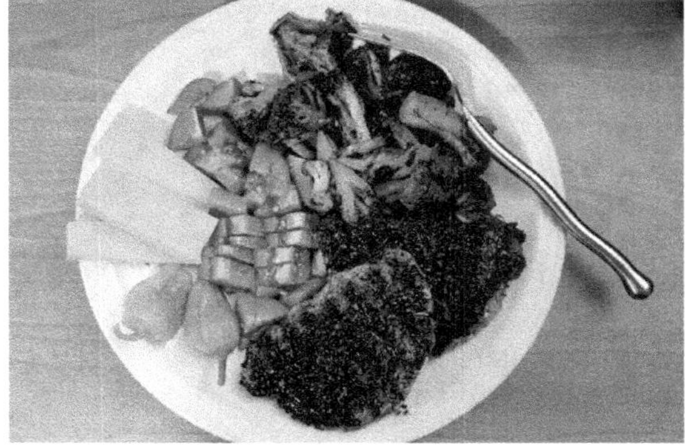 flashed with a few ounces of white wine. After the wine reduce by 80%, I added a bit of lemon juice, then soy sauce, took it from the heat, and tossed it with a tablespoon of butter.

The tomatoes were covered in olive oil, balsamic vinegar, and sea salt.
Rounding off the plate with extra sharp, cheddar cheese and a few pepperoncini led to a very satisfying meal.

Roast Chicken, Sundried Tomatoes, in Cream Sauce

This was an experiment in making a heavy cream substitute from butter and half-n-half that costs 70% less than using heavy cream. It works reasonably well.

Gently melt 1/6 cup unsalted butter in the microwave and pour into 7/8 cup of half-n-half. Do this in a plastic container with a tight-fitting lid and shake the heck out of it and it will emulsify. Use, heat, and reduce the same way as regular heavy cream.

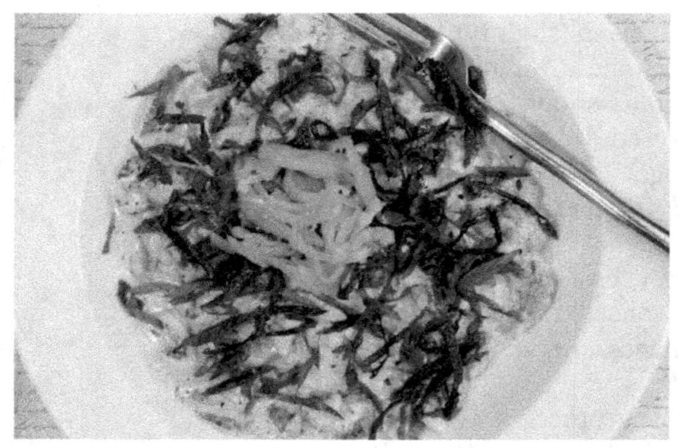

Side Note: Reducing/reduction is heating the cream, or other liquid, at a boil, to reduce its volume and thicken it. So, you'll often see recipes tell you to "reduce by half" or "reduce by a third". The further something is reduced, the closer you need to watch it. It's easy to reduce a liquid to nothing and suddenly burn your food.

For this dish I took left over chicken legs (see below), pulled the meat from the bones, and cut into bite sized pieces (after removing any cartilage and tendon). Placed into a hot pan (wok) with a bit of olive oil, brought up to high temp, then added a few ounces of white wine, which I reduced by 2/3rds.

When the white wine was reduced, I added the pseudo-heavy cream and, while that was reducing at a very strong simmer, finished heating zoodles in the microwave, and, after pouring off the water, added them to the chicken and cream mix.

It continued to reduce to a slightly loose consistency (so the cream would coat the back of a spoon, but nowhere near as thick as honey). I lowered the temperature and added parmesan cheese to help thicken it. (If, after a minute, it isn't thick enough, add a little more cheese. If it is too thick, add a little milk or water.)

After plating, I topped it with slices of sundried tomatoes, sliced green onion, and sliced pepperoncini.

Sausage and Greens

A simple dish of mixed, spring greens tossed with olive oil, balsamic vinegar, and salted/peppered to taste served with bratwurst straight from the cast iron, grilling pan, sundried tomatoes, pepperoncini, and sharp, cheddar cheese.

Simple, easy, and satisfying.

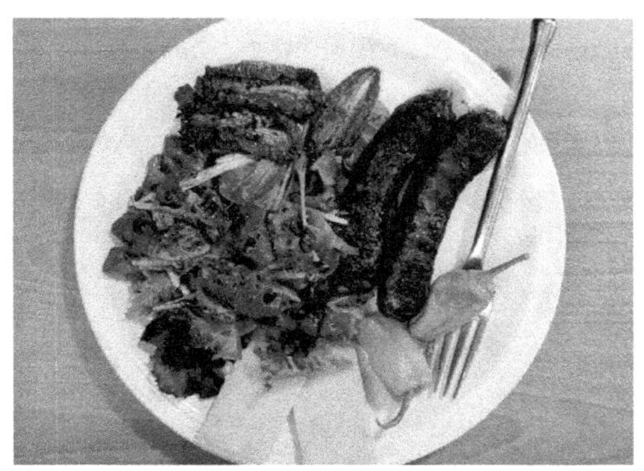

Sausage, Tomatoes, and Zoodles

This is zoodles, made from yellow squash, cooked in the microwave to al dente, tossed with a little bit of olive oil, and then plated.

On top of that are two (precooked) sliced bratwurst sautéed in olive oil, then an added

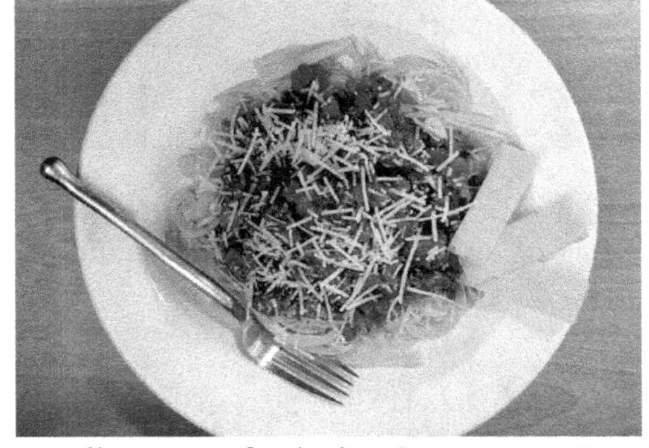

can of drained, diced tomatoes, with a small amount of red wine. Parmesan on top of that, some sharp, cheddar on the side, and you have a simple, nourishing meal.

This is an example of dry brining. I wanted to see if the salt, and flavors, would work their way through the skin into the meat.

They did.

Each side of the chicken legs were first lightly covered in medium grind sea salt, then crushed red pepper, then dried Italian seasoning mix.

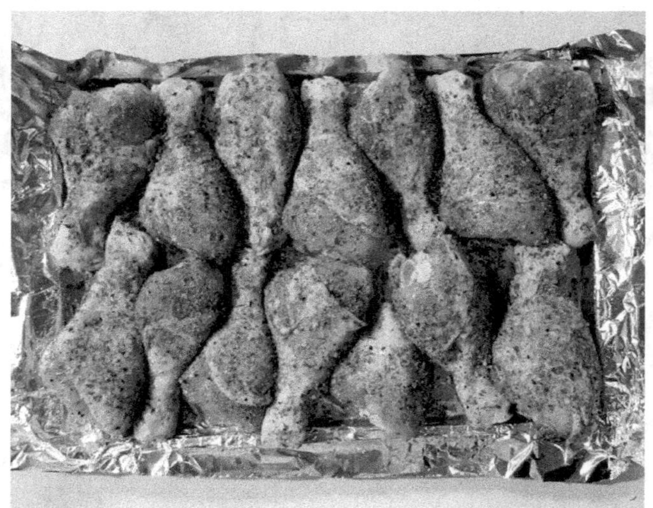

They sat covered in the fridge for 18 hours and the pieces were turned a few times.

Baking at 425 F, for 40 minutes, and turning them at 30 minutes, resulted in very juicy chicken with crispy skin. A meat thermometer inserted near the bone, at the fat end, read 165 F—which is the temp you want your chicken to get to.

So, there you have it, a few techniques, a few ideas, and a few examples of what I eat on a low carb diet. All of this can be applied to the foods you like to eat and in the proportions you enjoy.

Don't be afraid to experiment.

Enjoy the journey!

--Evan

An Assortment of Lower Carb Vegetables (values are grams per 1 cup)

	Carbs	Sugar	Fiber	Net Carbs
Kale	0.9	0.2	0.9	0.0
Watercress	0.4	0.1	0.2	0.2
Lettuce (red leaf)	0.6	0.1	0.3	0.3
Lettuce (green leaf)	1.0	0.2	0.5	0.5
Lettuce (romaine)	1.5	0.6	1.0	0.5
Spinach	1.0	0.1	0.7	0.3
Arugula	0.7	0.4	0.3	0.4
Swiss Chard	1.3	0.4	0.6	0.7
Bok Choy	1.5	0.8	0.7	0.8
Mustard Greens	2.6	0.7	1.8	0.8
Celery	3.0	1.3	1.6	1.4
Cucumber	1.8	0.8	0.3	1.5
Mushrooms (white)	2.2	1.3	0.7	1.5
Mushroom (portabella)	3.3	2.2	1.1	2.2
Mushroom (Cremini)	3.7	1.5	0.5	3.2
Radish	3.9	2.1	1.9	2.0
Eggplant	4.8	2.8	2.5	2.3
Asparagus	5.2	2.5	2.8	2.4
Summer Squash	3.7	2.4	1.2	2.5
Zucchini	3.8	3.1	1.2	2.6
Bell Peppers (green)	4.2	2.2	1.6	2.6
Cabbage	5.1	2.8	2.2	2.9
Cauliflower	5.3	2.0	2.1	3.2
Bean Sprouts	4.0	0.0	0.5	3.5
Broccoli	6.0	1.5	2.4	3.6
Fennel	6.3	3.4	2.7	3.6
Green beans	6.9	3.2	2.7	4.2
Okra	7.4	1.4	3.2	4.2
Brussels sprouts	7.8	1.9	3.3	4.5
Scallions, chopped	7.3	2.3	2.6	4.7
Tomato	7.0	4.7	2.2	4.8
Turnips	8.3	4.9	2.3	6.0
Carrots	12.2	6.0	3.6	8.6
Leek	12.5	3.4	1.6	10.9
Onion, chopped	14.9	6.7	2.7	12.2
Pumpkin	20.0	10.0	6.1	13.9

Fat Content of select meats (per 100 grams):

	Fat (g)
Pork Belly	53.0
Pork bacon	49.0
Prime rib	33.7
Beef ribs	28.1
Lamb ribs	25.3
Pork rib	23.9
Beef short rib	22.6
New York strip	22.1
Pork shoulder	21.4
Lamb chops	21.2
T-bone	20.4
Ground lamb	19.7
Rib eye	19.0
Ground turkey	17.5
Ground beef	17.4
Filet mignon	17.1
Ground bison	15.1
Top sirloin	14.2
Lamb burger	14.0
Dark meat chicken	13.8
Lean ground beef	12.0
Lean ground turkey	11.6
Veal	11.4
Pork loin	11.1
Ground chicken	10.9
Pork loin	8.8
Flank steak	8.2
Turkey	7.4
Beef chuck	6.8
Extra lean gr beef	5.5
Ham	5.1
Pork tenderloin	4.0
Skinless chicken brst	3.6
Extra lean gr turkey	2.7
Venison	2.4
Turkey breast	2.1

Fat Content of select cured meats (per 100 grams):

	Fat (g)
Pepperoni	46.3
Bacon & Beef Sticks	44.2
Chorizo	38.3
Kielbasa	29.6
Bratwurst	29.1
Cheesefurter	29.0
Pâté	28.4
Knackwurst	27.7
Scrapple	26.0
Bockwurst	25.9
Liver Cheese	25.6
Mortadella	25.4
Frankfurter	24.6
Bologna	24.4
Salami	24.0
Beerwurst	21.3
Corned Beef	14.9

Grams of Carbs, Fat & Protein in Selected Cheeses (per ounce/28 grams):

	Carbs	Fat	Protein
Blue Cheese	0.7	8.2	6.1
Brie Cheese	0.1	7.9	5.9
Camembert	0.1	6.9	5.6
Cheddar Cheese	0.9	9.5	6.5
Cheddar Sharp	0.6	9.5	6.8
Colby Cheese	0.7	9.1	6.7
Cottage Cheese	1.0	4.9	3.2
Cottage Cheese NF	1.9	0.3	3.0
Cottage Cheese (2%)	1.4	2.6	3.0
Edam Cheese	0.4	7.9	7.1
Feta Cheese	1.2	6.0	4.0
Goat Cheese hard	0.6	10.0	8.7
Goat Cheese soft	0.0	6.0	5.3
Gouda Cheese	0.6	7.8	7.1
Gruyere Cheese	0.1	9.2	8.5
Monterey Cheese	0.2	8.6	7.0
Parmesan	0.9	7.3	10.2
Provolone Cheese	0.6	7.6	7.3
Ricotta Cheese	0.9	16.1	3.5
Romano Cheese	1.0	7.7	9.0
Swiss Cheese	0.4	8.8	7.7

Checklists

On my journey to get and stay lean:

- I consistently tried to…
    o **ELIMINATE SUGAR** from my diet
    o **LOWER CARBS** to about 20 grams/day
    o **EAT MORE FAT** (saturated and monounsaturated)
    o **READ NUTRITION/INGREDIENT LABELS** on food to check net carbs and sugar content
    o **AVOID SNACKING**
    o **AVOID SUGARY DRINKS**
    o **EXERCISE 20 MINUTES A DAY** (even just walking) 5 days/week
- Sometimes I…
    o Would eat more than 20 grams of carbs a day—like at a party, while on vacation or celebrating a special occasion; then I'd get back to LCHF.
- I learned…
    o To be sure to **eat enough**—when I ate too little (I was trying to lose weight!) I was always tired and didn't lose as much weight
    o To **eat more fat**: This was difficult because all my life I'd heard fat was bad for you
    o The difference between various types of fats and to **stay away from seed oils** (soy oil, sunflower oil, corn oil) **and trans fats**
    o To really **watch my carb intake**—it's easy for it to creep up over time because they are hidden in most processed foods, and they are tasty
    o To **eat more salt** because on a low-carb/high-fat diet, you pee out more of the salt you eat; and research shows that we need between 2 and 4 grams of salt a day—which is more than the current recommended daily amount. I take a supplement of sodium and magnesium every few days.
    o To listen to my body—**to stop eating when full and only eat when hungry** (I stopped eating out of habit)
    o To **trust the approach** even if my weight plateaued for a few weeks